Orthopaedics and Rheumatology

on the move

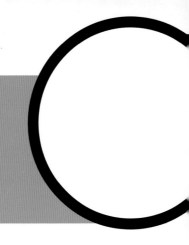

Orthopaedics and Rheumatology
on the move

Authors: **Terence McLoughlin, Ian Baxter, Nicole Abdul**
Editorial Advisor: **Andrew Hamer**

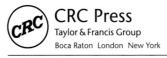

CRC Press
Taylor & Francis Group
Boca Raton London New York

CRC Press is an imprint of the
Taylor & Francis Group, an **informa** business

First published in 2013 by
CRC Press
Taylor & Francis Group
6000 Broken Sound Parkway NW, Suite 300
Boca Raton, FL 33487-2742

© 2013 McLoughlin, Baxter, Abdul
CRC Press is an imprint of Taylor & Francis Group, an Informa business
No claim to original U.S. Government works
Printed and bound in India by Replika Press Pvt. Ltd.
Version Date: 20120813
International Standard Book Number: 978-1-444-14567-0
1 2 3 4 5 6 7 8 9 10

Visit the Taylor & Francis Web site at
http://www.taylorandfrancis.com
and the CRC Press Web site at
http://www.crcpress.com

Cover images © Sebastian Kaulitzki – Fotolia & © franckreporter/istockphoto.com (smartphone)

Contents

Preface

Have you ever found orthopaedics and rheumatology overwhelmingly complicated? Are you simply short of time and have exams looming? If so, this short revision guide will help you. Written by students and junior doctors, this book presents information in a wide range of formats including flow charts, summary tables and authentic images annotated with comments. During the course of writing this book, the students among us have now become qualified doctors ourselves.

Orthopaedics and rheumatology are important specialties for any clinician as they encompass a myriad of commonly seen conditions in both the acute and chronic settings. This book has been designed to be used by medical students and junior doctors 'on the move', both on the wards and as essential preparation for exams.

No matter what your learning style, we hope you will find this book appealing and easy to read. We think that this innovative style will help you, the reader, to connect with this often feared topic – helping you to learn and understand it (maybe even enjoy it!) while also helping to prepare you for exams and life as a junior doctor.

We of course welcome your feedback on how this book measures up and how you feel it could aid your study and work better. Everyday is a new learning experience for us all.

Authors:

Terence McLoughlin BSc MBChB – Foundation Year 2 doctor in academic research, The Royal London Hospital, North East London Deanery, UK
Ian Baxter BMedSci MBChB – Foundation Year 1 doctor in medical education, The Northern General Hospital, Yorkshire and the Humber Deanery, UK
Nicole Abdul BMedSci MBChB – Foundation Year 2 doctor, The Northern General Hospital, Yorkshire and the Humber Deanery, UK

Editorial advisors:

Andrew Hamer Consultant Orthopaedic Surgeon, The Northern General Hospital, Sheffield, UK

We would like to thank Dr Andrew Keat for his advice regarding the rheumatology component of the book, and Miss Caroline Blakey for her invaluable input in reviewing and refining our initial draft.

EDITOR-IN-CHIEF:

Rory Mackinnon BSc MBChB – GP Trainee Year 1, Queen Elizabeth Hospital, Gateshead, UK

SERIES EDITORS:

Sally Keat BMedSci MBChB – Foundation Year 2 doctor, Northern General Hospital, Sheffield, UK
Thomas Locke BSc MBChB – Foundation Year 2 doctor, Northern General Hospital, Sheffield, UK
Andrew Walker BMedSci MBChB – Specialist Trainee Year 2 Doctor in Medicine, Northern General Hospital, Sheffield, UK; also author of chapter 14, Vasculitides.

Acknowledgements

Thank you to all the additional contributors, particularly Miss Alison Baxter for medical illustrations.

The authors would also like to thank their friends and families for all their support and patience during medical school and the start of our careers.

List of abbreviations

- ABCDE: airway, breathing, circulation, disability, exposure
- ABPI: Ankle brachial pressure index
- AC: Acromioclavicular
- ACL: Anterior cruciate ligament
- ACR: American College of Rheumatologists
- ALP: Alkaline phosphatase
- ANA: Antinuclear antibodies
- ANCA: Anti-neutrophil cytoplasmic antibodies
- anti-CCP: Anti-cyclic citrullinated peptide
- AP: Anteroposterior
- AS: Ankylosing spondylitis
- ASIS: Anterior superior iliac spines
- ATLS: Advanced trauma life support
- AVN: Avascular necrosis
- BMD: Bone mineral density
- BMI: Body mass index
- CK: Creatine kinase
- CPPD: Calcium pyrophosphate dihydrate
- CRP: C-reactive protein
- CSF: Cerebrospinal fluid
- CT: Computed tomography
- DDH: Developmental dysplasia of the hip
- DIP: Distal interphalangeal
- DM: Diabetes mellitus
- DMARDs: Disease-modifying antirheumatic drugs
- DRE: Digital rectal examination
- DVT: Deep vein thrombosis
- DXA: Dual energy x-ray absorptiometry
- ESR: Erythrocyte sedimentation rate
- FBC: Full blood count
- FSH: Follicle-stimulating hormone
- GCA: Giant cell (temporal) arteritis
- GCS: Glasgow Coma Scale
- GGT: Gamma-glutamyl transpeptidase
- GI: Gastrointestinal
- HGPRT: Hypoxanthine guanine phosphoribosyl transferase
- HLA: Human leukocyte antigen
- HSP: Henoch–Schönlein purpura

- IBD: Irritable bowel disease
- IVDU: Intravenous drug user
- JVP: Jugular venous pressure
- LCL: Lateral collateral ligament
- LFTs: Liver function tests
- LH: Luteinizing hormone
- LMN: Lower motor neurone
- LOSS: Loss of joint space, osteophytes, sclerosis and subchrondral cysts
- MC&S: Microscopy, culture and sensitivity
- MCL: Medial collateral ligament
- MCP: Metacarpophalangeal
- MDT: Multidisciplinary team
- MI: Myocardial infarction
- MRI: Magnetic resonance imaging
- MTP: Metatarsophalangeal
- MUA: Manipulation under anaesthesia
- NICE: National Institute for Health and Clinical Excellence
- NOF: Neck of femur
- NSAIDs: Non-steroidal anti-inflammatory drugs
- OA: Osteoarthritis
- ORIF: Open reduction, internal fixation
- OSCE: Objective structured clinical examination
- PA: Posteroanterior
- PAN: Polyarteritis nodosa
- PCL: Posterior cruciate ligament
- PE: Pulmonary embolism
- PERLA: Pupils equal and responsive to light and accommodation
- PET-CT: Positron emission tomography-computed tomography
- PIP: Proximal interphalangeal
- PMR: Polymyalgia rheumatica
- PPI: Proton pump inhibitor
- PSA: Prostate specific antigen
- RA: Rheumatoid arthritis
- RF: Rheumatoid factor
- RTA: Road traffic accident
- SLE: Systemic lupus erythematosus
- SOCRATES: Site, onset, character, radiation, associated findings, timing, exacerbating/relieving factors, severity
- SUFE: Slipped upper femoral epiphysis
- TB: Tuberculosis
- TED: Thromboembolus deterrent
- TENS: Transcutaneous electrical nerve stimulation

- U&Es: Urea and electrolytes
- UC: Ulcerative colitis
- UMN: Upper motor neurone
- USS: Ultrasound scan
- WCC: White cell count
- WHO: World Health Organization

An explanation of the text

The book is divided into three parts: orthopaedics (upper limb and lower limb), rheumatology, and a self-assessment section. We have used bullet points to keep the text concise and brief and supplemented this with a range of diagrams, pictures and MICRO-boxes (explained below).

Normal range values are given for most tests in this book as a guideline for your knowledge. Please note that ranges differ between laboratories and therefore you should always use figures from your own institution to interpret results.

MICRO-facts

These boxes expand on the text and contain clinically relevant facts and memorable summaries of the essential information.

MICRO-print

These boxes contain additional information to the text that may interest certain readers but is not essential for everybody to learn.

MICRO-case

These boxes contain clinical cases relevant to the text and include a number of summary bullet points to highlight the key learning objectives.

MICRO-reference

These boxes contain references to important clinical research and national guidance.

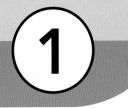

General principles and fracture management

1.1 OVERVIEW

Please refer to Chapter 4, Shoulder, for a comprehensive formula for joint history and examination. To avoid repetition, we will not include the same information in every chapter.

1.2 FRACTURES

DEFINITION

- A fracture is an abnormal interruption of the cortex of a bone.
- Fractures can be closed (simple) or open (compound):
  - Closed: skin surface remains intact.
  - Open: skin or visceral surface is broken, resulting in a higher risk of infection.

AETIOLOGY

- Trauma: the type of fracture is related to the mechanism of injury and the forces applied.
- Pathological: the underlying bone is abnormal and fails more readily.
- Repetitive stress can lead to a stress fracture.

CLASSIFICATION

- There are numerous classification systems used in orthopaedics.
- As a medical student it is not necessary to learn them all, however you should know about two in particular:
  - Salter-Harris classification for paediatric fractures (see Chapter 10, Ankle and foot)
  - Gardner classification of hip fractures (see Chapter 8, Hip).

> **MICRO-facts**
>
> The mechanism of injury affects the forces applied to bones and the resulting fracture configuration.

- Tension = transverse fracture including avulsion injuries
- Bending = triangular fracture
- Compression = short oblique fracture
- Twisting = spiral fracture
- Classifications are based on fracture location, displacement and number of fragments involved (Table 1.1).
  - The general principles of fracture management are to bring the two ends of the broken bones into close proximity.
  - This allows callus formation and bone healing in a functional and anatomical position.
  - Consequently, pain is alleviated and functional state optimized.
  - Reduce, immobilize, rehabilitate.
    - **Reduce**: correct the displacement by appropriate manipulation.
    - **Immobilize**: strapping, splinting, cast, internal and external fixation.
    - **Rehabilitate**: early mobilization, physiotherapy, occupational therapy and social support.

Note: it is important to encourage smoking cessation and adequate nutritional intake to assist bone healing.

If the patient requires surgical intervention as part of their fracture management, the following principles are important to consider:

- **Important pre-operative considerations**:
  - Obtain informed consent and optimize the patient.
  - Nutritional status (but remember to keep the patient nil by mouth prior to surgery if having general anaesthetic).
- **Fluid balance**
  - Correct any coagulopathy.
  - Appropriate investigations completed.
  - Consider venous thromboembolic prevention.

Table 1.1 Describing a fracture.

INFORMATION NEEDED	DESCRIPTION
Bone involved	May sound obvious, but very important to mention
Site of fracture	Proximal, diaphyseal and distal
Displacement	Translation (shift), rotation (twist), angulation (tilt), length (shortening). The distal segment is described in relation to the proximal segment
Number of fragments involved	2 = simple >2 = comminuted

- **Important intra-operative considerations**:
  - Aseptic conditions
  - Good surgical technique
  - Minimize blood loss (use of tourniquet and diathermy)
  - Maintain fluid balance
  - Prophylactic antibiotics, if indicated.
- **Important post-operative considerations**:
  - Venous thromboembolic prevention (early mobilization, adequate hydration, thromboembolus deterrent (TED) stockings, low molecular weight heparin)
  - Regular physiotherapy
  - Optimize nutritional status.

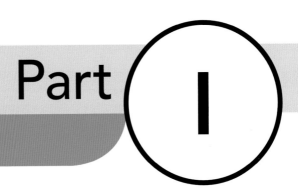

Part I

Upper limb

2 Head and neck

2.1 OVERVIEW

Head and neck injuries can vary from minor to the catastrophic. An understanding of head and neck pathology is essential in managing emergency, as well as elective situations (Fig. 2.1). This chapter describes some of the more common head and neck injuries and orthopaedic pathology that might be encountered.

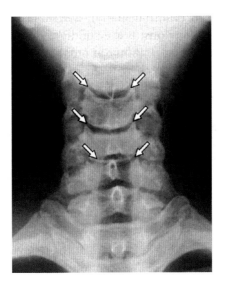

Fig. 2.1 Basic anatomy of the head and neck. **Imaging – normal x-rays (a)** Anteroposterior view – note the smooth, symmetrical outlines and the clear, wide uncovertebral joints (arrows). **(b)** Open mouth view – to show the odontoid process and atlanto-axial joints. **(c)** Lateral view – showing all seven cervical vertebrae. Reproduced with permission from Solomon L, Warwick D, Nayagam S. *Apley's System of Orthopaedics and Fractures*, 9th edn. London: Hodder Arnold, 2010.

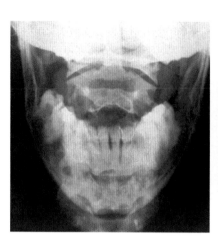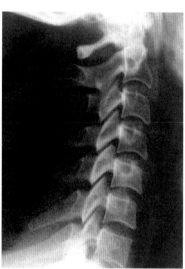

Fig. 2.1 (*Continued*)

2.2 HISTORY

> **MICRO-facts**
>
> A supporting history from a witness is essential if the patient is confused or unconscious.

DEMOGRAPHICS

What are the age and occupation of the patient?

PRESENTING COMPLAINTS

Follow the SOCRATES (site, onset, character, radiation, associated findings, timing, exacerbating/relieving factors, severity) pain assessment

- Site
- Onset:
    - When did it start?
    - How did it start?
- Character: describe the pain: is it sharp/dull/aching?
- Radiation. Does the pain radiate? If so does it correspond to a known dermatome(s)?

- Associated findings: Is there stiffness, instability, clicking, grinding, catching, weakness, pins and needles?
- Timing. Is the pain worse at a particular time of day?
- Exacerbating/relieving factors: Are there positions that increase/improve symptoms?
- Severity. Out of 10 how bad is the pain?

ASSESS IMPACT OF THE PAIN

- How does it affect coping at home/leisure activity and work.
- Is the pain unchanged or has there been progression in the level of disability?

HISTORY OF PRESENTING COMPLAINT

- Has the same pain/problem occurred previously?
- Has the patient received previous treatment for the presenting problem?
- If so how was it treated?

PAST MEDICAL HISTORY

- Has the patient suffered any previous trauma?
- Has the patient undergone previous surgery?
- Are there any previous medical conditions?

2.3 HEAD AND NECK EXAMINATION

MICRO-facts

Reminder of general trauma examination principles:
- Secure the C spine
- Primary survey: airway, breathing, circulation, disability, exposure (ABCDE)
- Take care with patient transfer as further cervical spine injury may be caused
- Secondary survey including a full neurovascular examination

INSPECTION

- Check for symmetry, muscle bulk, wasting, scars.
- Abnormal neck contour, signs of trauma.

PALPATION

- Feel for local muscle/bony tenderness, especially posteriorly; deformities (particularly the neck 'step' sign).

Upper limb

MOVEMENT

- Is cervical spine injury suspected? Start with active movements. Elicit the full range of movement. Ask patient to perform the following movements and note range.
- First active then passive (normal range in brackets):
  - Forward flexion
  - Backward extension
  - Lateral ('ear to shoulder')
  - Rotation ('shake head')
- Repeat the same range with passive movements.

GLASGOW COMA SCALE

The Glasgow Coma Scale (GCS) is the initial part of assessing the trauma patient. Regular reassessment of GCS is an essential determinant as to the severity of the head injury and indicates whether the patient is deteriorating or improving. The GCS score is on a scale of 15: alert, 15/15; severe injury, <8/15; unresponsiveness, 3/15 (Table 2.1).

Table 2.1 **Glasgow Coma Scale.**

MOTOR RESPONSE (6)	VERBAL RESPONSE (5)	EYE OPENING (4)
6. Obeys commands		
5. Localises to pain	5. Orientated	
4. Withdraws to pain	4. Confused	4. Spontaneous
3. Flexes to pain	3. Inappropiate	3. Open to speech
2. Extends to pain	2. Incomprehensible	2. Open to pain
1. No response to pain	1. None	1. No response

MICRO-facts

When assessing the eyes, examine the pupils. Are pupils equal and responsive to light and accommodation (PERLA)?
With increased intracranial pressure the third nerve may be compressed causing non-reactive pupil dilatation.

2.4 IMPORTANT HEAD PATHOLOGY

FACIAL FRACTURES

Mechanism of injury

Head pathology is usually caused by a direct blow to the face.

Anatomy

The bones most usually affected are the zygomatic arch, maxilla and mandible.

Assessment

- Facial fractures are usually treated by a specialist maxillofacial team. In the Emergency Department (ED), the primary diagnosis of facial fractures will often come within the remit of the orthopaedic surgeon.
- The Le Fort classification is used for facial fractures. There are three Le Fort types of fracture (Table 2.2).

Table 2.2 Le Fort classification.

LE FORT I	LE FORT II	LE FORT III
Nose intact	Fracture across nose	Fracture across nose
Orbits intact	Medial orbital fracture	Lateral orbital fracture
Maxilla fracture	Middle third of face mobile	

> **MICRO-facts**
>
> If the maxilla is unstable, it may become depressed and obstruct the airway.

Management

Depending on the severity of the fracture, the maxillofacial team may manage the injury with plating of the fracture to give it greater support.

HEAD INJURIES

Mechanism of injury

Head injuries are caused by trauma to the head and neck either by a direct blow or indirect force.

Assessment

Assessment should be divided into those associated with or without a skull fracture and the secondary or resulting brain pathology:

- Cerebral oedema
- Brain contusion/laceration
- Vascular injury (extradural/subdural haemorrhage/thrombosis) (Fig. 2.2) and
- The consequential clinical effects: GCS; ante/retrograde amnesia; neurological deficit: late effects, e.g., post-traumatic epilepsy/personality change

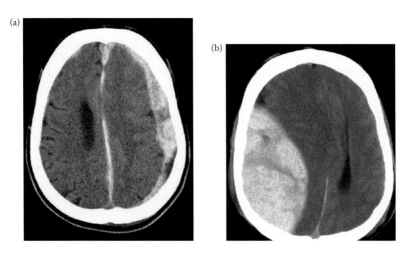

Fig. 2.2 Extradural haematoma (a) subdural haematoma (b). Reproduced with permission from Solomon L, Warwick D, Nayagam S (eds.). *Apley's System of Orthopaedics and Fractures*, 9th edn. London: Hodder Arnold, 2010.

Continuous assessment of GCS is mandatory. Useful localizing clinical signs of a skull fracture can be found in the MICRO-facts box.

MICRO-facts

Head injury signs
- Frontal fossa: raccoon eyes; subconjunctival haemorrhage (without a margin)
- Middle fossa: cerebrospinal fluid (CSF)/blood rhinorrhoea/otorrhoea
- Posterior fossa: Battle's sign

NECK FRACTURES

Hangman's fracture
Mechanism of injury and anatomy
- Fracture of the C2 pedicle (through the pars interarticularis)
- Caused by distraction and hyperextension of the cervical spine
- For assessment and management, see below under Management.

MICRO-print
If you suspect a basal skull fracture, you must avoid using nasopharyngeal airways to secure the airway as there is a (very small) chance you may enter the skull rather than the upper airway.

Mid-cervical fractures

Mechanism of injury and anatomy

- Fracture of C3, 4 and/or C5 spine.
- Often as a consequence of catastrophic trauma.
  - Examples include road traffic accidents, horse riding accidents and contact sports, such as martial arts and rugby.
  - If the fracture occurs at C3, 4 or 5, breathing as well as other functions may be compromised.
  - Remember C3, 4, 5 roots comprise the components of the phrenic nerve which controls diaphragmatic movement ('C3, 4, 5, keeps the diaphragm alive').

Assessment

- C-spine control must be present at all times (Advanced Trauma Life Support (ATLS) protocol)
- Spinal x-rays in more than two planes (anteroposterior (AP), lateral and 'peg') + computed tomography (CT) scan of the head and neck are the current gold standard of assessing the severity of C-spine fracture.

Management

- Immobilize C-spine
  - Urgent neurosurgical involvement
  - Depending on severity and neurological impairment: from conservative to urgent neurosurgical intervention
  - Neurorehabilitation involving a multidisciplinary team (MDT) may be indicated.
    - In severe cases, this stage of management may occur over many months in a spinal injuries unit.

DISC PROLAPSE

MICRO-case

A previously fit 52-year-old male presented to the Emergency Department complaining of a 1-week history of sudden collapse. He was a ship's captain. His history was of sudden upper and lower limb weakness and falling whenever he bent down or looked up into a mirror while shaving. He had no loss of consciousness and no post-ictal symptoms.
Cervical spine x-ray series showed a C2 or Hangman's fracture.

Points to consider

- Hangman's fracture was causing episodic transient tetraplegia on acute flexion/extension of neck while shaving.
- The fracture had occurred 1 week before during a storm at sea when he had been thrown across his cabin. There was no remembered history of trauma during this event.

Mechanism of injury

- Prolapse of the intervertebral cervical disc is usually caused by sudden flexion and/or rotation of the neck.
- There is often a background of cervical spondylosis.

Assessment

Results in disc protrusion with:
- Neck pain due to compression of the posterior longitudinal ligament, and/or
- Arm pain/paraesthesia due to foraminal nerve root compression.
- Nerve roots most commonly involved: C5/6 and 7.

Management

- Depends on the severity of the symptoms – from conservative to surgical intervention
- Central disc prolapse is a surgical emergency.

CERVICAL SPONDYLOSIS

Mechanism of injury

- Common degenerative arthropathy. Symptoms usually begin from age 40 years, increasing with age.

Anatomy and assessment

- Often asymptomatic
- May present as intermittent pain and stiffness extending from the occiput to the scapulae
- Pathology: Degenerative disc collapse; bony spurs with exit foramen nerve root compression
- X-rays may or may not show osteoarthritic change.

Management

Management is commonly conservative with physiotherapy and analgesia, as required.

RHEUMATOID ARTHRITIS

- See Chapter 11, Rheumatoid arthritis.
- Thirty per cent of rheumatoid arthritis patients have atlanto-axial erosion (C1/C2 level).
- This may lead to subluxation of the joint.

- Symptoms include pain and restricted neck movement.
- Upper motor neurone (UMN) signs may be present if there is cord compression.

MICRO-print
X-ray of the rheumatoid cervical spine might look severe.
While it is rare for serious consequences to occur, it is imperative that appropriate x-rays are available to the anaesthetist if the patient is to have a general anaesthetic.

Upper limb

3 Thoracic and lumbar spine

3.1 OVERVIEW

Disorders of the thoracic and lumbar spine form an important part of orthopaedics. Back pain is the most common presenting symptom. Conditions may range from being a mild irritation to the patient, through to medical emergencies, such as cauda equina syndrome. Careful history taking and examination is necessary to determine the cause and severity of the problem.

3.2 BASIC ANATOMY OF THE SPINE

Fig. 3.1 shows the anatomy of the thoracic and lumbar vertebrae.

SPINE HISTORY

The most common presenting complaints of patients with disorders of the spine include:
- Pain
- Stiffness
- Deformity.
  Key points of the history which must be covered include:
- Asking about the timing of the symptoms as this can give clues as to the origin of the problem. If it is worse at rest, then think about osteoarthritis of the spine. If worse after exercise, then it is most likely to be due to soft tissues such as the musculature and ligaments supporting the spine.
- Constant boring, nagging pain with a band distribution around the torso, which is present at night should raise the possibility of a malignant or infective cause.
- Has the patient noticed a deformity?
- Is there any numbness or paraesthesia in any of the limbs? What dermatomal nerve distribution are these in? This might indicate nerve root compression.
- Is bladder and bowel function and sensation normal? Any retention, incontinence or altered sensation may indicate a possible cauda equina syndrome, which is a medical emergency.

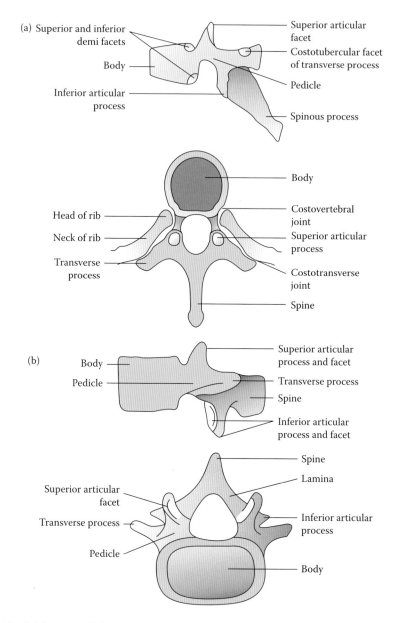

Fig. 3.1 Diagram of thoracic vertebrae (a); diagram of lumbar vertebrae (b); dermatome diagram (c); myotome diagram (d). Reproduced with permission from Abrahams P, Craven J, Lumley J, *Illustrated Clinical Anatomy*, 2nd edn. London: Hodder Arnold, 2011.

(c)

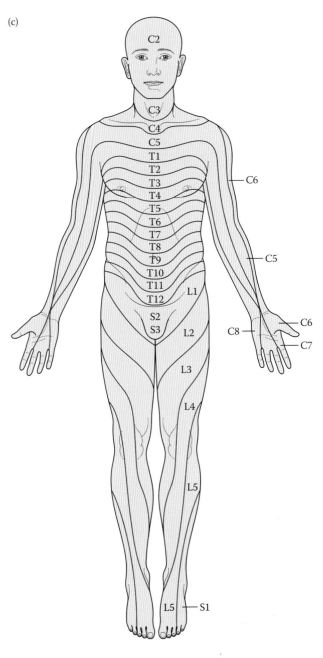

Fig. 3.1 (*Continued*)

(d)

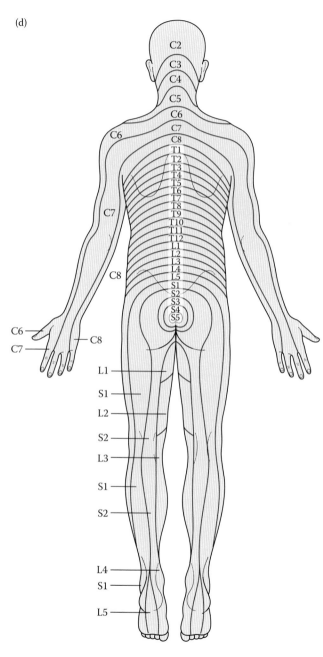

Fig. 3.1 (*Continued*)

EXAMINATION OF THE BACK

Look

- Observe the patient's normal gait and posture.
- With the patient standing, inspect the patient from the back, side and from the front.
- While assessing from behind, look for any asymmetry, muscle wasting or scoliosis.
- When looking from the side, the shape of the patient's spine can be assessed. Things to look for from the side are:
  - Cervical lordosis
  - Thoracic kyphosis
  - Lumbar lordosis
- A chest wall deformity may be seen from the front in certain conditions.
- Look for café-au-lait spots: six or more are suggestive of neurofibromatosis, which is associated with scoliosis and kyphosis.
- Hairy patches at the base of the spine may also be seen which suggest spina bifida.

Feel

- Feel down the spinal processes and over the sacroiliac joints. It is important to note any abnormal differences between vertebrae.
- During the examination, it should be identified whether the patient's pain originates from either the bony vertebrae or the surrounding soft tissue (e.g. the paraspinal muscles and ligaments).

Move

- Ask the patient to lean forward to touch their toes to assess lumbar flexion. If you place two fingers on the lumbar spine, these should move apart on flexion and together on extension, when the patient leans backwards.
- Ask the patient to run one hand down the outside of their leg to assess lateral flexion. Repeat on the other side and compare.
- With the patient standing, leg power can be assessed by asking the patient to first take a couple of steps on their tip toes (assessing plantar flexion) and then on their heels (assessing dorsiflexion).
- Thoracic rotation can be assessed with the patient sitting on the couch. Place your hands on the patient's shoulders to guide the movement, ensuring both directions are observed.
- With the patient lying flat on an examination couch, a straight leg raise test can be performed. This is a test for lumbosacral nerve root tension. The leg is raised until the patient experiences pain in the buttock, thigh and calf (sciatic nerve pain). The angle that is achieved is noted. Patients should be able to raise the leg to 80–90°.
- Finally, upper and lower limb neurological examinations should be carried out.

Upper limb

MICRO-facts

If there is any suspicion from the history that the patient has cauda equina syndrome, then a rectal examination checking for tone and perianal sensation must be performed.

IMAGING THE SPINE

- Any initial imaging is likely to consist of an anteroposterior and lateral radiograph of either the thoracic or lumbar spine.
- Computed tomography (CT) is a useful method for identifying structural bone changes and disc prolapse. The development of three-dimensional images of the spine allows surgeons to gain a clear idea of the patient's spinal structure.
- Magnetic resonance imaging (MRI) gives a very clear picture of the structure of the spine and is very useful for looking at the soft tissues in the back (Fig. 3.2). It is used to visualize the spinal canal and cord, intervertebral discs as well as the vertebral bodies.

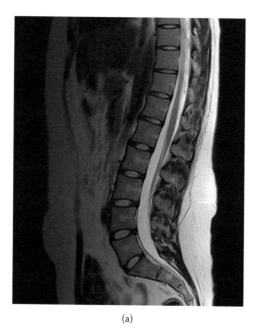

(a)

Fig. 3.2 Magnetic resonance image (MRI) of a normal spine (a); MRI showing a prolapsed intervertebral disc (b). Reproduced with permission from Abrahams P, Craven J, Lumley J, *Illustrated Clinical Anatomy*, 2nd edn. London: Hodder Arnold, 2011.

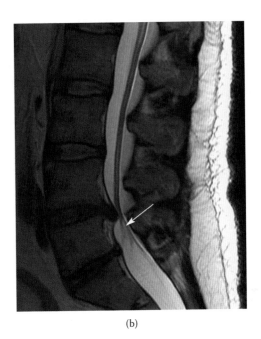

(b)

Fig. 3.2 (*Continued*)

3.3 SCOLIOSIS

DEFINITION

Scoliosis is an apparent lateral curvature of the spine and deformity is the usual presenting feature.

AETIOLOGY AND PATHOPHYSIOLOGY

- The cause of the vast majority of cases is unknown.
- Scoliosis most commonly occurs in girls and a thoracic curve, convex to the right, is most frequently seen.
- There are two broad categories of scoliosis:
    - **Postural scoliosis**: this is an apparent scoliosis often due to a leg length discrepancy. This disappears on sitting.
    - **Structural scoliosis**: this is defined as a lateral angulation of the spine of >10° with rotation of the vertebrae. Structural scoliosis can be further subdivided into:
        - Congenital and infantile
        - Neuromuscular
        - Metabolic.
    - Idiopathic adolescent scoliosis is the most common type of scoliosis, occurring in 90% of cases.

CLINICAL FEATURES

A posterior abdominal hump or a rib hump secondary to the rotational aspect of the scoliosis is the most visible sign of scoliosis.

INVESTIGATIONS

- The angle of the curve is measured on the full length standing posteroanterior (PA) spine radiograph and is called Cobb's angle.
- Lateral spine radiographs will enable assessment of kyphosis and lordosis.
- Gait assessment.
- True and apparent leg length measurements.
- Full neurological examination, including looking for the appearance of hairy patches, haemangiomas or lipomas in the lumbar region of the spine which may indicate spina bifida.

MANAGEMENT

- Progression of the curve is not inevitable and in cases where the Cobb angle is less than 20° (Fig. 3.3), spontaneous resolution may occur. In most cases, progression of the curve accelerates at times of growth particularly during the growth spurt around the age of puberty.
- It is important to take into account the patient's potential for further growth when deciding upon treatment. The patient's age, time since menarche and radiographic parameters, such as Risser's staging (Fig. 3.4) are all important factors for establishing whether a child is likely to have reached skeletal maturity.

TREATMENT

- The aims of treatment are to either stop a curve from progressing further or to correct an existing curve.
- Treatment methods include:

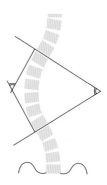

Fig. 3.3 Measuring the Cobb angle. The angle of curvature is measured on the x-ray by Cobb's method: Lines projected from the top of the uppermost and the bottom of the lowermost vertebral bodies in the primary curve define Cobb's angle. Reproduced with permission from Solomon L, Warwick D, Nayagam S. *Apley's System of Orthopaedics and Fractures*, 9th edn. London: Hodder Arnold, 2010.

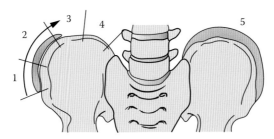

Fig. 3.4 Risser's staging of skeletal maturity. Grade 1 is given when the ilium (bone) is calcified at a level of 25%; it corresponds to prepuberty or early puberty. Grade 2 is given when the ilium (bone) is calcified at a level of 50%; it corresponds to the stage before or during growth spurt. Grade 3 is given when the ilium (bone) is calcified at a level of 75%; it corresponds to the slowing of growth. Grade 4 is given when the ilium (bone) is calcified at a level of 100%; it corresponds to an almost cessation of growth. Grade 5 is given when the ilium (bone) is calcified at a level of 100% and the iliac apophysis is fused to iliac crest; it corresponds to the end of growth. Reproduced with permission from Solomon L, Warwick D, Nayagam S (eds.). *Apley's System of Orthopaedics and Fractures*, 9th edn. London: Hodder Arnold, 2010.

- Corrective casting: this is done in infantile idiopathic scoliosis and may prevent the scoliosis from progressing.
- Bracing: there are several different braces in use and it remains a controversial method of treatment. They aim to stop progression of the scoliosis.
- Surgery: this may be needed in severe and worsening curves when the patient cannot tolerate the cosmetic deformity.
- Surgical treatment involves a posterior spinal fusion in combination with spinal instrumentation. It is a major operation with potentially severe risks including spinal cord injury, which could result in paraplegia.

MICRO-case

A 14-year-old girl presents in your follow-up scoliosis clinic. She has been monitored over the past few years and despite trying a brace, her Cobb angle is now 52° and she is not happy with how her back looks and it is causing her pain. It is decided that surgery is the most appropriate option.

Points to consider
- The Cobb angle is the maximal angle of the primary curve.
- Defining features of scoliosis are a lateral angulation of the spine of >10° with rotation of the vertebrae.

3.4 KYPHOSIS

DEFINITION

Although kyphosis is the normal convexity seen in the thoracic spine, an exaggeration of this norm (>45°) is still known as a kyphosis.

AETIOLOGY AND PATHOPHYSIOLOGY

- Kyphosis is associated with a change in shape in several of the thoracic vertebrae.
- There are many different causes for a kyphosis and they are most easily grouped by the ages at which they affect the individual.
- Causes for a child with a kyphosis include:
  - Congenital vertebral defect
  - Achondroplasia
  - Osteogenesis imperfecta
  - Tuberculosis
  - Muscular dystrophy
  - Polio.
- In adolescents, the most common cause is Scheuermann's disease:
  - Anterior wedging of the vertebrae occurs due to a failure in the thoracic vertebral bodies to grow as they should.
  - Scheuermann's disease is still not fully understood.
  - Boys are affected more than girls and they often complain of backache and fatigue.
  - Treatment remains controversial as to whether bracing is effective, however, curves of less than 40° do not require treatment.
- In the elderly, the most common cause is due to degeneration of the intervertebral discs with slight wedging of some of the thoracic vertebral bodies.
  - This can lead to a kyphosis which if the patient suffers a wedge fracture of the thoracic spine as a result of osteoporosis can be much more noticeable and painful.
  - Treatment is with analgesia and if osteoporosis is found to be the cause, then bisphosphonates and calcium replacement should be given, as necessary.

CLINICAL FEATURES

Curvature of the spine is best seen with the patient side on.

INVESTIGATIONS

Investigations are tailored to a suspected cause, but anteroposterior (AP) and lateral radiographs are important for measuring the curvature.

MANAGEMENT

- Management is dependent on cause, severity and patient wishes.
- Treatment options include monitoring, medical treatment with a brace and a multitude of surgical options dependent on the severity and nature of the kyphosis.

- The characteristic stoop of an elderly woman with a kyphosis is called a 'dowager's hump'. Although they may be present, vertebral fractures are not required for the kyphosis to develop.
- The term is not eponymous. Dowager is a noun which refers to any elderly woman, especially one who is wealthy or behaves with dignity.

3.5 SPINAL INFECTION

BACTERIAL DISCITIS

Bacterial discitis is bacterial infection of the vertebral disc

Aetiology and pathophysiology

- Acute spinal infection is uncommon and in its early stage may be difficult to diagnose.
- It is more common in children.
- Infection usually occurs due to haematogenous spread from a distant site or through the introduction of bacteria during an invasive procedure on the spine.
- *Staphylococcus aureus* is the most common causative organism.
- Diagnosis is achieved by CT-guided biopsy sent for culture.

Clinical features

- Patients will have constant severe back pain with C-reactive protein (CRP).
- Patients are often afebrile and systemically well.
- Affected children will poorly tolerate spinal flexion.
- Neurological deficit may be present.

Investigations

- Blood cultures
- AP and lateral radiographs looking for disc space narrowing.
- Using CT scan, it is possible to detect discitis at an earlier stage and also identify paraspinal disease.
- MRI scan is the most sensitive and specific test for discitis and therefore rules out other differentials.
- Biopsy.

Management

- Prolonged course of intravenous antibiotics (6–8 weeks) based on organism sensitivities
- Immobilization with a brace.

Upper limb

SPINAL TUBERCULOSIS

Definition

- Extrapulmonary tuberculosis affecting the spine, also known as Pott's disease.
- The spine is the most common musculoskeletal site for tuberculosis (TB) infection.

Aetiology and pathophysiology

- Caused by various strains of mycobacterium, but most commonly *Mycobacterium tuberculosis.*
- It is an uncommon condition in the UK, however, it is still a large problem elsewhere in the world.
- Nonetheless, the incidence in the UK is increasing due to the numbers of immunosuppressed individuals, as well as increased drug resistance.
- It results from haematogenous spread from other affected sites (pulmonary TB is most common).
- Seeding of infection occurs within the subchondral bone of the anterior inferior endplate.

Clinical features

- The clinical picture is of a slow onset back pain with longstanding ill health.
- There may also be neurological signs relevant to the level of disease (Pott's paraplegia).
- Symptoms include fever, night sweats and weight loss.

Investigations

- Elevated inflammatory markers e.g. C-reactive protein (CRP)
- Mantoux skin test (will be positive)
- MRI of the spine
- CT-guided biopsy for acid-alcohol fast bacilli (AAFB) and TB culture

Management

- Treatment is with antituberculosis chemotherapy (RIPE: rifampicin, isoniazid, pyrazinamide and ethambutol).
- Surgical drainage of any abscess may be required.

3.6 ACUTE PROLAPSE OF AN INTERVERTEBRAL DISC

DEFINITION

Acute prolapse of an intervertebral disk is defined by herniation of the nucleus pulposus through the annulus fibrosus.

AETIOLOGY AND PATHOPHYSIOLOGY

- Most commonly affects active, well individuals and may be associated with heavy exercise.
- The most commonly involved discs are:
  - L5/S1 (which is the most common)
  - L4/L5
  - L3/L4
- The intervertebral discs consist of a nucleus pulposus at the centre that is surrounded by the annulus fibrosus.
- During an intervertebral disc prolapse there is rupture of the annulus. This allows the nucleus to protrude posteriorly.

CLINICAL FEATURES

- The protrusion usually bulges to one side of the posterior longitudinal ligament producing pain in the buttock, posterior thigh and calf (sciatica) and the patient will have a restricted straight leg raise on the affected side.
- If the nerve root is directly compressed, then the patient will also suffer from paraesthesia and numbness in the relevant dermatomal distribution along with weakness and depressed reflexes in the myotome.

INVESTIGATIONS

- Perform straight leg raise to test for sciatic pain.
- Plain radiographs have a limited role in showing the soft tissues, however, they are useful in identifying other pathology such as tumours.
- MRI provides the optimal soft tissue images.
- If neurological deficit is suspected, then nerve conduction studies or an electromyogram can be useful.

MANAGEMENT

- Analgesia, such as non-steroidal anti-inflammatory drugs (NSAID) may be useful in the acute phase, and maintaining gentle exercise is important.
- Most symptoms will settle in 6–8 weeks with conservative measures.
- Surgery is indicated if:
  - Conservative treatment fails, i.e. neurological symptoms progress.
  - Symptoms of cauda equina syndrome are present.
- Rehabilitation following resolution of symptoms is vital to prevent future attacks.

COMPLICATIONS

- If, as occurs rarely, the rupture of the annulus is large and central then the protruding nucleus may press on the cauda equina. This is a medical emergency and can produce the following symptoms:
  - Painless retention of urine
  - Urinary incontinence

Upper limb

- Faecal incontinence
- Perianal anaesthesia
- Bilateral sciatica
- Lower limb weakness.

- Patients with suspected cauda equina lesions need an urgent MRI to identify the level of the problem before going to theatre for surgical decompression, as otherwise the patient can be left severely disabled.

MICRO-print

If the cause of the symptoms is a tumour pressing on the cauda equina, high-dose corticosteroids, such as dexamethasone, can be given prior to surgery. The steroid reduces the swelling in and around the cauda equina, which may be contributing to compression. This is a very effective adjunct to surgical treatment and reduces the chance of the patient becoming paralysed.

3.7 SPINAL STENOSIS

This occurs due to narrowing of the spinal canal, often due to the degeneration of the spine vertebrae seen with ageing.

- Symptoms include vague backache, as well as pain, weakness and paraesthesia in the legs. Patients often complain that their problem is worse on standing than sitting.
- Symptoms may be very similar to those seen in intermittent claudication and as such is sometimes called spinal claudication.

MICRO-case

Mrs Radian is a 75-year-old right-handed retired cook. She presents to the fracture clinic after falling over while out walking her dog a week ago. She says that at the time of the accident when she felt herself falling she put her right hand out in front of her to break the fall, subsequently breaking a bone. She does recall that after the fall her hand and wrist oddly made a 'dinner fork' shape and her wrist was painful. It now causes her no bother but the cast around it is somewhat cumbersome! From the information Mrs Radian has given, you realize she had a distal radial fracture (Colles' fracture).

Points to consider
- Distal radial fractures are common in elderly post-menopausal women.
- Falling on an outstretched hand is a common mechanism for sustaining a Colles' fracture.
- The 'dinner fork' shape that the patient reports her hand and wrist made is the result of dorsal displacement of the distal radius.

3.8 SPONDYLOLISTHESIS

Spondylolisthesis means a slipped vertebra. It involves the forward displacement of one vertebral body on the vertebra below. It most commonly occurs between the L5/S1 or L4/L5 vertebral bodies. It can be due to osteoarthritis (elderly) or a congenital defect in the pars interarticularis (young adults).

TREATMENT

Either conservative or surgical treatment may be appropriate.

MICRO-case

An overweight 65-year-old woman goes to her GP complaining of pain in both of her calf muscles when she walks more than 50 metres. It is worse when walking downhill. The pain has come on over the past few months. It completely settles when she sits down to rest. On examination, you find she has good strong foot pulses and her legs are warm.

Given that this woman appears to have intact vascular supply to her legs, intermittent claudication is less likely to be the cause but would be high on your list of differentials. The diagnosis in this case is spinal stenosis likely caused by vertebral degeneration.

Points to consider

- Spinal stenosis is caused by narrowing of the spinal canal.
- It is important to ask about symptoms of pain, weakness and paraesthesia as these will all aid your diagnosis.
- Intermittent claudication is the most likely alternative diagnosis, so a careful vascular history and examination should be performed.

3.9 THORACIC AND LUMBAR SPINE FRACTURES

MECHANISM OF INJURY/AETIOLOGY

- Thoracolumbar fractures can be caused by the following:
  - Insufficiency fractures: low-energy fractures occurring in osteoporotic bone
  - Burst fractures
  - High energy: the vertebral column may fracture if exposed to significant twisting and flexion forces.
- Vertebral fractures of the thoracic spine are relatively uncommon as they are further stabilized by the rib cage.
  - When they do occur, there is a greater risk of neurological damage as the spinal canal is relatively narrow.
  - This means that when damage does occur, it is usually complete.

Upper limb

- There are three main pattern types of vertebral fracture:
  - Flexion
  - Extension
  - Rotation.
- Below the level of L1 is the cauda equina and so with fractures occurring below this level it is the lower nerve roots that are at risk.
- Plain x-rays are useful for viewing the lower thoracic and lumbar vertebrae, however, the ribs and scapulae make visualization of the upper thoracic vertebrae difficult.
- CT is the best option for imaging especially as rapid sequencing CT is available. MRI is useful for assessing soft tissue and neurological injuries.

CLINICAL FEATURES

- Moderate to severe back pain, which is worse on mobilization.
- If there is spinal cord involvement, then there may be symptoms of numbness, tingling and incontinence or urinary retention.

TREATMENT

- Dependent on the fracture pattern seen and stability of the fracture, fractures may be managed conservatively with a brace or require surgical stabilization.
- The main aims of surgery are to sufficiently reduce the fracture, relieve pressure on the spinal cord and nerves and allow the patient to mobilize as early as possible.

COMPLICATIONS

- As patients are immobile following a vertebral fracture they are at risk of developing a deep vein thrombosis (DVT) or pulmonary embolism (PE).
- If depth of breathing is insufficient, patients are at risk of developing pneumonia.
- Careful management of pressure areas is needed to reduce the risk of pressure sores occurring.

Upper limb

4 Shoulder

4.1 OVERVIEW

Movement of the shoulder involves the glenohumeral joint and the acromioclavicular joint, as well as movement between the scapula and the posterior chest wall (scapulothoracic movement). The basic anatomy of the shoulder is described in Fig. 4.1.

4.2 SHOULDER HISTORY

DEMOGRAPHICS

- Age
- Occupation
- Is the patient left or right handed?

PRESENTING COMPLAINTS

Presenting complaints include the SOCRATES (site, onset, character, radiation, associated findings, timing, exacerbating/relieving factors, severity) pain assessment.

- Site
- Onset: When did it start? How did it start?
- Character: describe the pain, e.g. sharp, dull, aching
- Radiation: does the pain radiate anywhere?
- Associations: e.g. stiffness, instability, clicking, grinding, catching, weakness, pins and needles
- Timing: is the pain worse at a particular time of day?
- Exacerbating/relieving factors: positions that worsen symptoms
- Severity: out of 10 how bad is the pain?

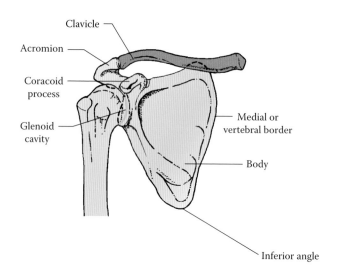

Clavicle

Acromion

Coracoid process

Glenoid cavity

Medial or vertebral border

Body

Inferior angle

Fig. 4.1 A diagram of the anterior view of the shoulder joint. Reproduced with permission from Clancy J, McVicar A. The skeleton. In: *Physiology and Anatomy for Nurses and Healthcare Practitioners. A Homeostatic Approach,* **3rd edn. London, Hodder Arnold, 2009: 79.**

ASSESS IMPACT OF THE PROBLEM

It is important to ask about the impact on daily function at home and work and to assess the progression of the problem:
- Can the patient put on a coat or fasten their bra?
- Combing the hair or lifting objects may be difficult.
- Is it getting worse, better or staying the same?

HISTORY OF PRESENTING COMPLAINT

- Has this problem occurred previously?
- Has the patient received any previous treatment for this problem? If so, what was the management?

PAST MEDICAL HISTORY

- Has the patient suffered any previous trauma?
- Has the patient undergone any previous surgery?
- Are there any medical conditions, e.g. ligamentous laxity?

FAMILY HISTORY

- Have other members of the patient's family had a similar problem?
- Is there a family history of ligamentous laxity or multidirectional instability of the shoulder?

Upper limb

4.3 SHOULDER EXAMINATION

See Table 4.1 for differential diagnosis of shoulder pain.

Table 4.1 Differential diagnosis for shoulder pain.

ROTATOR CUFF	GLENOHUMERAL JOINT	SCAPULOTHORACIC	REFERRED PAIN
Tendonitis/ subacromial bursitis	Osteoarthritis	Muscle injury	From neck
Rotator cuff tear	Rheumatoid arthritis	Subscapular bursitis	Diaphragmatic pain (shoulder tip)
Rupture of long head of biceps	Septic arthritis	Long thoracic nerve (winging)	Apical lung cancer
Acromioclavicular joint subluxation/ dislocation	Instability/ dislocation	Myeloma/bone metastases	Brachial plexus lesion
	Myeloma/bone metastases		

REMINDER OF GENERAL EXAMINATION PRINCIPLES

- Explain beforehand to the patient what you are doing.
- Do not cause undue pain or discomfort.
- Examine the joint above and below.
- Compare sides.

INSPECTION

- General symmetry, muscle bulk, wasting and scars
- Abnormal shoulder contour/loss of deltoid bulk (suggestive of anterior dislocation)
- Abnormal clavicular contour (clavicle and acromioclavicular (AC) joint)
- Winging of the scapula
- Never forget the axilla!

PALPATION

- Never forget temperature! Use the back of your hand.
- Palpate along full joint line: sternoclavicular to AC joint to scapula. Feel for deformity and tenderness.

Upper limb

MOVEMENT

- Start with active movement: elicit full joint range in the patient. Ask the patient to perform the following movements and note range (normal range in brackets):
  - Abduct each arm (0–170°: 0–90° = glenohumeral; 90–170° = scapulothoracic)
  - Forward flexion (0–165°)
  - Backward extension (0–60°)
  - Elbows at 90°, tucked into side. External (0–70°) and internal rotation
  - Composite movements to assess functionality: Hand behind the head (with elbow fully back). Hand behind the back (try to touch contralateral scapula).
- Repeat movements passively, (feeling over the joint for crepitus)
- Special tests performed against resistance:
  - Rotator cuff
    - Supraspinatus: test abduction starting with arm by the side
    - Infraspinatus/teres minor: test external rotation with arm in neutral position
    - Subscapularis: test internal rotation with hand behind back pushing examiner's hand away
  - Scapula: Get patient to press hands against wall and assess for winging (Fig. 4.2).

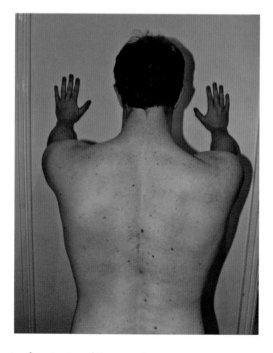

Fig. 4.2 Assessing for winging of the scapulae.

4.4 COMMON SHOULDER PATHOLOGY

SUBLUXATION AND DISLOCATION OF THE ACROMIOCLAVICULAR JOINT

Mechanism of injury and anatomy

- Caused by fall onto lateral aspect of the shoulder forcing the acromion downwards.
- In subluxation, the capsule is torn but the conoid and trapezoid ligaments are intact.
- In dislocation, both the capsule and ligaments are torn and the acromion is displaced markedly downwards.
- It is much more common than sternoclavicular joint injury.
- It is a common injury in rugby players.

Assessment

- Clinical examination and x-rays (see Figs 4.3, 4.4 and 4.5).

(a)

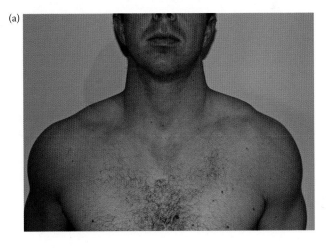

Fig. 4.3 (a–c) Acromioclavicular joint injury.

Upper limb

(b)

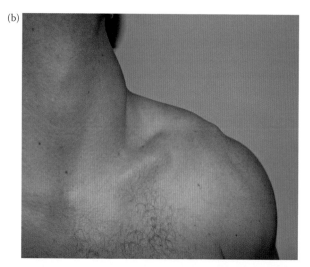

(c)

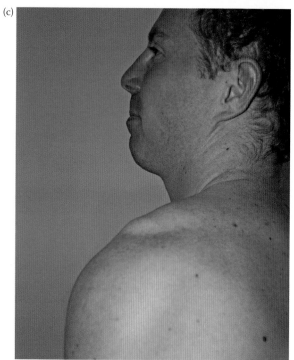

Fig. 4.3 (*Continued*)

(a)

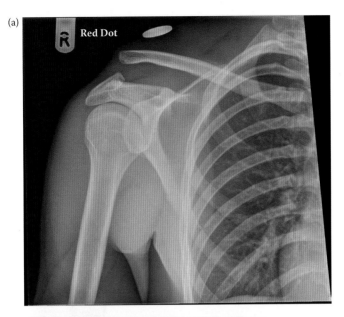

(b)

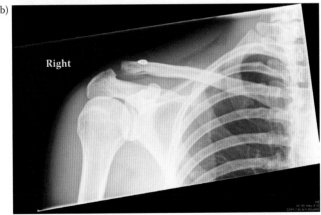

Fig. 4.4 (a) Complete disruption of the acromioclavicular joint. (b) Post-operative x-ray following surgical repair.

MICRO-facts

Note the asymmetry seen between the left and right shoulder. A subtle but definite step can be seen over the AC joint caused by the 'sprung' clavicle.

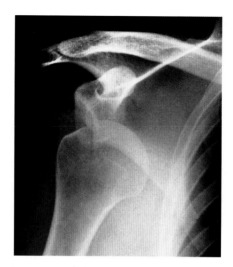

Fig. 4.5 X-ray showing anterior dislocation of the shoulder. Reproduced with permission from Solomon L, Warwick D, Nayagam S (eds.). *Apley's System of Orthopaedics and Fractures,* 9th edn. London: Hodder Arnold, 2010.

Management

- Subluxation: conservative ± sling for 2 weeks. Encourage early shoulder rehabilitation.
- Dislocation: conservative + sling for 2–4 weeks.
- Even gross instability has a good outcome.
- Surgical internal fixation with a screw is possible, but complications are common and risks may outweigh benefit.

ANTERIOR DISLOCATION OF THE SHOULDER

Mechanism of injury

- Common due to shallow glenohumeral joint space plus large range of movement (Fig. 4.6).
- Caused either by fall on outstretched hand or by forced abduction and external rotation of the shoulder.

Assessment

- Patient often presents with holding injured arm by other hand across the chest.
- Sudden severe pain with loss of deltoid bulk and a small bulge may be palpated below the clavicle.

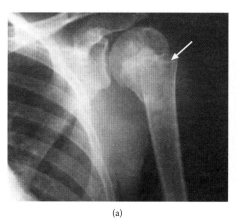

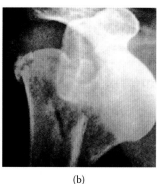

(a)   (b)

Fig. 4.6 (a) X-ray showing a fractured humeral head. Reproduced with permission from Abrahams P, Craven J, Lumley J. The upper limb. In: *Illustrated Clinical Anatomy.* London: Hodder Arnold, 2011 (b) X-ray showing anterior fracture dislocation of the humerus. Reproduced with permission from Solomon L, Warwick D, Nayagam S (eds.). *Apley's Concise Orthopaedics and Fractures,* 9th edn. 2010 London: Hodder Arnold, 2010.

MICRO-facts

Always check for an associated fracture of the proximal humerus, particularly if the mechanism of injury is high impact.

Always check and record the neurovascular status of the arm both before and after reduction of the joint, in particular the axillary nerve (the 'regimental badge' distribution on the deltoid).

Management

- First, rule out a fracture prior to reduction.
- Four reduction methods: manipulation under anaesthesia (MUA), hanging arm, Hippocratic and Kocher methods:
  - Manipulation under general anaesthesia.
  - Hanging arm: pronate patient and let arm hang off bed freely. May require intravenous pethidine or diazepam for muscle relaxation.
  - Hippocratic: gently but firmly pull the arm away from patient while the body is in counter-traction. Used when muscle relaxation cannot be achieved by hanging arm method.
  - Kocher: involves slow external rotation of the flexed arm to relax the subscapularis muscle and then the arm is raised and rotated medially.
- Place arm in sling and repeat x-ray to assess joint position.

> **MICRO-print**
> **Post-reduction complications**
> Rotator cuff tear, nerve injury (axillary nerve), vascular injury (axillary artery), and recurrent dislocation (if glenoid labrum has been damaged).

MICRO-facts

Note that a posterior shoulder dislocation is rare but commonly missed on anteroposterior (AP) x-ray. Clinically, the arm will be locked in medial rotation.

Have a high index of suspicion in patients following an epileptic fit or electrocution.

MICRO-case

A 19-year-old male rugby player attends a walk-in centre after playing in a rugby match and being side tackled on his right. He is holding his left arm over his torso. He is in considerable pain. On examination, there is a loss of deltoid bulk. A clinical diagnosis of anterior shoulder dislocation was confirmed on shoulder x-ray.

Points to consider

- An anterior shoulder dislocation was due to traumatic fall.
- Relocation of a shoulder can be by MUA, hanging arm, Hippocratic and Kocher methods.
- Axillary nerve palsy is a possible complication causing sensory loss in the regimental badge distribution causing

FRACTURES OF THE PROXIMAL HUMERAL HEAD

Mechanism of injury

Fractures of the proximal humeral head are caused by a fall onto an outstretched hand.

Assessment

- Usually occur after middle age.
- Occur most frequently in osteoporotic individuals.
- Fractures classified in terms of affected site (surgical neck, anatomical neck, greater or lesser tuberosity) and the number of fragments. Neer's classification is most commonly used.
- Impacted fractures (seen as a dense line on x-ray, see Fig. 4.5) are more common than displaced fractures.

- Extensive bruising to the area may be seen, though this may occur later.
- Diagnosis confirmed by x-ray.
- Axillary nerve or brachial plexus injury should be considered.

Management

- If impacted or minimally displaced, a short period of rest in a sling (2–3 weeks) is recommended.
- Active movement is encouraged as soon as is practical, but care must be taken to prevent disimpaction of the fracture.
- If the fracture is displaced or severely angulated then open reduction and internal fixation may be required.

MICRO-print

Humeral head fractures in the setting of a shoulder dislocation are difficult to manage. Closed reduction may still be possible, but when there is a large degree of displacement, an open procedure may be necessary.

MICRO-case

A 38-year-old female presents to the Emergency Department with a painful upper left arm after tripping over a pavement onto her outstretched arm. Of note in her history is a body mass index (BMI) of 19, which has been the case since she was 16 years old.

Points to consider

- There are many risk factors for osteoporosis apart from post-menopause and in this case there is a possibility of low bone density due to:
  - Low weight
  - Nutritional deficiency/anorexia
  - Dysmennorrhea

5 Elbow

5.1 OVERVIEW

The elbow is a synovial hinge joint between the distal humerus and proximal radius and ulna (Fig. 5.1).

Flexion and extension, along with supination and pronation enable us to move our hands to our mouths and head, reach areas on our backs, carry objects, as well as being important for when we are working both while sitting down and standing.

ELBOW EXAMINATION

Inspection

- Ensure both arms are fully exposed.
- Ask the patient to stand with their arms by their sides, elbows fully extended with palms facing forward. Look at the symmetry of the two sides, muscle bulk of the biceps and forearms, scars, psoriatic plaques, obvious swelling.

(a)

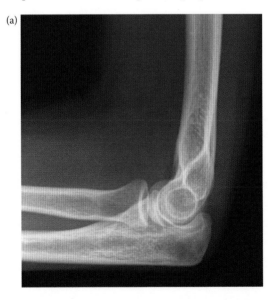

Fig. 5.1 Basic anatomy of the elbow. X-ray, lateral view. Reproduced with permission from Abrahams P, Craven J, Lumley J. *Illustrated Clinical Anatomy*, 2nd edn. London: Hodder Arnold, 2011.

(b)

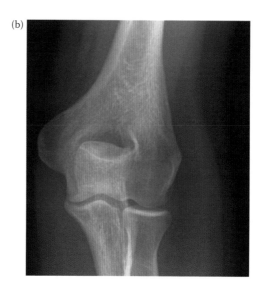

(c)

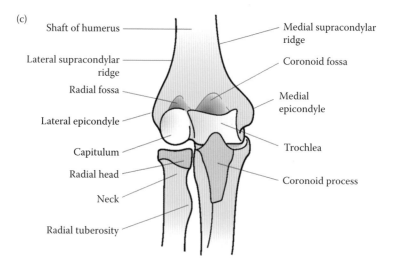

Shaft of humerus

Lateral supracondylar ridge

Radial fossa

Lateral epicondyle

Capitulum

Radial head

Neck

Radial tuberosity

Medial supracondylar ridge

Coronoid fossa

Medial epicondyle

Trochlea

Coronoid process

Fig. 5.1 (*Continued*)

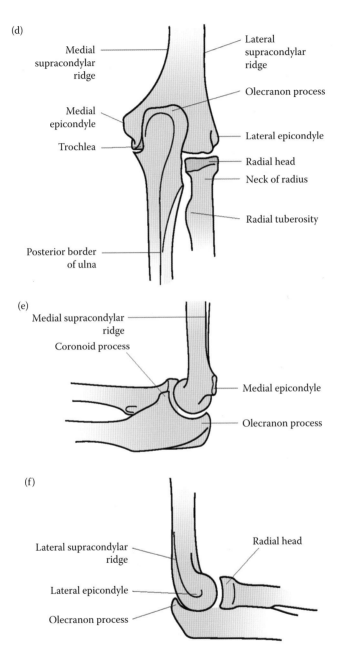

(d)

Medial supracondylar ridge

Lateral supracondylar ridge

Olecranon process

Medial epicondyle

Trochlea

Lateral epicondyle

Radial head

Neck of radius

Radial tuberosity

Posterior border of ulna

(e)

Medial supracondylar ridge

Coronoid process

Medial epicondyle

Olecranon process

(f)

Lateral supracondylar ridge

Radial head

Lateral epicondyle

Olecranon process

Fig. 5.1 (*Continued*)

Palpation

- Never forget to feel the temperature of the skin, using the back of your hand.
- With the elbow flexed to 90°, palpate the olecranon, medial and lateral epicondyles, joint line and the head of the radius.
- Feel for swelling of the joint and assess for any fluctuance, as well as for rheumatoid nodules and tenderness.

Movement

Start with active movement. Elicit the full joint range in the patient.

- Ask the patient to perform the following movements and note range (normal range in brackets):
  - Elbow flexion to extension (140–0°) some patients, particularly young girls, may hyperextend their elbows though this is entirely normal.
  - Elbow pronation (palm down) (90° from mid position).
  - Elbow supination (palm up) (90° from mid position).
  - Composite movements to assess functionality: Ask the patient to move each hand to their mouth and to touch behind their head and back.
- Repeat all these movements passively, noting any crepitus.
- It is important to also examine the patient's cervical spine and shoulder, as problems with these joints commonly cause pain that is referred to the elbow.
- Examination of the hand is also important to assess for neurological signs as a result of elbow pathology.

5.2 COMMON ELBOW PATHOLOGY

With the patient in the anatomical position, the arms are slightly abducted at the elbow. This is known as the 'normal carrying angle' and the normal range is between 5 and 15°.

CUBITUS VALGUS

- Cubitus valgus is when the carrying angle of the elbow is greater than the normal 5–15°.
- It is an acquired deformity, most commonly after a malunion of a lateral condylar fracture.

CUBITUS VARUS

Definition

Cubitus varus is when the carrying angle is decreased.

Aetiology

It is most commonly seen following a malunion of a supracondylar fracture.

Clinical features

The deformity may be known as a gunstock deformity due to its appearance. It is most easily seen when the shoulder is abducted with the elbow extended.

Treatment

Correction of both cubitus valgus and varus is by osteotomy.

TENNIS ELBOW (LATERAL EPICONDYLITIS)

Definition

Tennis elbow is characterized by gradual onset of tenderness over the lateral epicondyle of the elbow. It most commonly occurs in active patients aged 30–50 years old.

Pain is due to a small tear, fibrosis, calcification or a vascular reaction in the tendon fibres of the common extensor origin.

Although tennis players may be affected, anyone who performs forceful gripping and wrist extension, such as while gardening, lifting or decorating, may be affected.

Diagnosis

- Diagnosis is made on the clinical history and examination. However, a plain x-ray may show sclerosis or calcification of the insertion.
- An ultrasound scan may be useful in assisting the diagnosis.

Management

- Treatment is by identification and adjustment of the causative activity, along with rest followed by physiotherapy. Anti-inflammatory medication may be helpful. Corticosteroid and local anaesthetic joint injection relieves symptoms, however it will not cure the problem.
- Most cases of tennis elbow will resolve in 6–12 months, but persistent symptoms may require surgical intervention.
- Surgery has a success rate of 80–85% and involves releasing the extensor tendon origin from the lateral epicondyle.

GOLFER'S ELBOW

- Golfer's elbow is similar to tennis elbow. However, it is much less common and causes pain over the medial epicondyle of the elbow.
- Pain most commonly due to a small tear in the tendon fibres of the common flexor origin (which insert on the medial epicondyle of the elbow).
- Diagnosis, investigations and management are the same as for tennis elbow, however treatment is less successful.

Upper limb

OLECRANON BURSITIS

Definition

Swelling of the olecranon bursa which is found lying over the ulna at the tip of the elbow (Fig. 5.2).

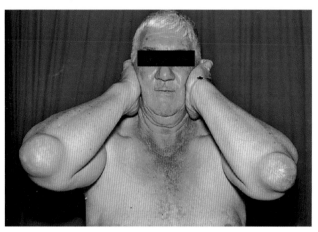

Fig. 5.2 Olecranon bursitis. Reproduced with permission from Solomon L, Warwick D, Nayagam S. *Apley's Concise System of Orthopaedics and Fractures*, 3rd edn. London: Hodder Arnold, 2005.

MICRO-case

Eleanor Bowe is a 64-year-old retired school teacher who now has time to dedicate to her true passion of gardening. However, last week she caught her elbow on a thorn while pruning her roses. Since then she has become unwell with a raised temperature and her elbow is swollen, warm and tender over the olecranon.

You suspect that this patient has septic olecranon bursitis most likely caused by *Staphyloccocus aureus* and so you take a joint aspirate for microscopy, cultures and sensitivities to confirm this before starting empirical intravenous flucloxacillin.

Points to consider

- Septic olecranon bursitis is caused by *Staphyloccocus aureus* in 40% of cases. Other significant organisms include *Streptococcus* sp. and less commonly Gram-negative bacilli.
- *S. aureus* grows as golden yellow colonies on blood agar with areas of haemolysis, and is coagulase positive.
- Always check the drug allergy status before starting any antibiotic.

Clinical features

Olecranon bursitis presents with a large swelling over the posterior aspect of the elbow. The elbow is likely to be warm but not always painful, depending on the cause and whether the bursitis is acute or chronic.

There are several causes of olecranon bursitis including the following:
- Repeated minor trauma, such as continual pressure or friction
- Gout
- Rheumatoid arthritis
- Infection

Investigations

- Routine blood tests can be performed to look for an underlying causative factor and to exclude an infection.
- Signs of rheumatoid arthritis or osteoarthritis may be visible on plain x-ray.

Management

- Management is dependent on the underlying cause.
- Simple and non-steroidal anti-inflammatory medications are first-line treatment.
- For persistently inflamed bursae, aspiration or surgical excision may be appropriate, but recurrence of swelling of the bursa is common.
- If infection is the cause of the bursitis, the most likely causative organism is *Staphylococcus aureus*. Therefore, empirical treatment with a penicillinase-resistant penicillin should be used, e.g. flucloxacillin. Always remember to check allergy status.
- Aim to start empirical antibiotics after you have taken an aspirate unless absolutely necessary. This will give you the best possible chance of identifying the pathogen.

LOOSE BODIES

Presentation

- Osteoarthritis
- Osteochondritis dissecans (devascularized bone segment which becomes loose)
- Acute trauma resulting in the loosening of a piece of cartilage
- The patient will complain of locking of the elbow joint limiting the range of various movements. This locking is commonly intermittent as the loose body floats around the joint.

Investigation

- A plain x-ray is useful for detecting the presence of any loose body and if further imaging is needed a computed tomography (CT) arthrogram may be helpful.

Upper limb

Management

- If the patient does not find their symptoms too distressing then they can be reassured and left alone.
- If the patient wishes to have them removed, this can be done either as an arthroscopic or open procedure.

OSTEOARTHRITIS

- This is likely to occur following trauma to the elbow joint or as a result of another underlying pathology, such as gout.
- The patient will present with pain and stiffness in the affected elbow. See Chapter 16, Non-inflammatory arthroses for more information.

RHEUMATOID ARTHRITIS

Rheumatoid arthritis is commonly bilateral and may affect both the elbow and superior radioulnar joint. It causes pain, swelling, tenderness, stiffness and instability of the elbow joint due to the destruction of the soft tissues which occurs.

- If pain is refractory to medical treatments (see Chapter 11, Rheumatoid arthritis):
- Excision of the radial head with a synovectomy
- Total elbow joint replacement.

MICRO-facts

Many of the pathologies in this chapter may cause the ulnar nerve to be compressed or stretched. The nerve lies in a groove behind the medial epicondyle passing through the cubital tunnel. It is here that it is at greatest risk of compression. The patient may present with a variety of neuropathic pathology in an ulnar nerve distribution.
Radial nerve compression may also occur, though this is rare.

5.3 TRAUMA

DISLOCATION OF THE ELBOW JOINT

Mechanism of injury/aetiology

- Relatively common injury sustained by both adults and children following a fall onto an outstretched hand.
- Posterior or posterolateral dislocation of the radius and ulnar are the most commonly seen elbow dislocations.

Clinical features

- Patient supporting their own arm in slight flexion.
- Olecranon and epicondyles are not in their usual anatomical position.
- There may be nerve damage which may be found on examination of the hand.
- Plain x-rays in at least two planes should be taken before an attempt at reduction of the dislocation is made so that all fractures are identified.

Treatment

- With an uncomplicated dislocation, reduction is with traction.
- Once reduced, the arm should be placed in a collar and cuff flexed at over 90° for 2 weeks after which time gentle mobilization can begin.

Complications

- As the elbow is usually a congruent joint, it is important that any associated fractures such as of the coronoid process, olecranon or radial head are also excluded.
- As with all dislocations and fractures, it is important that a neurovascular assessment is made and documented.

MICRO-print
Post-reduction complications of a dislocation or fracture dislocation of the elbow

- Damage to the brachial artery ± possibility of compartment syndrome
- Median or ulnar nerve injury (may recover in 6–8 weeks.)
- Stiffness with loss of some degree of extension (up to 30° is common)
- Myositis ossificans
- Recurrent dislocation.

MICRO-case

Oliver Cranon is a 23-year-old keen rollerblader. While at the skate park, he attempted a new trick off a jump that went wrong and he fell onto an outstretched arm. Fortunately, he was wearing wrist guards, but his elbow is in a great deal of pain and his friends were alarmed by his odd looking elbow.

This man is given analgesia and having examined him fully, plain x-rays reveal a posterior/posterolateral dislocation of the ulno-humeral joint due to fall on to his outstretched arm.

continued...

continued...

You inspect the x-rays carefully for evidence of any associated fractures before reducing the dislocation. On discharge you advise the patient of potential complications of his injury.

Points to consider

- It is important to examine the arm fully as the impact can cause fractures at any level right up to the clavicle.
- Associated fractures include fractures of the radial head, coronoid process or olecranon process.
- Late complications include stiffness with reduced range of motion, myositis ossificans or recurrent dislocation.

FRACTURES AFFECTING THE ELBOW

Supracondylar fractures of the distal humerus

- These are common fractures in children following a fall on an outstretched hand, but also occur less commonly in adults.
- There is a significant risk of neurovascular damage:
  - Brachial artery ± compartment syndrome
  - Median nerve.
  - A reduction in extension is almost certain and stiffness of the elbow joint is a common complication.

INTRA-ARTICULAR FRACTURES

Mechanism of injury/aetiology

These are normally as a result of high energy trauma to the elbow though they may occur in osteoporotic individuals with a simple fall.

Clinical features

- Swelling and deformity of the elbow
- Tenderness
- Reduced movement at the elbow joint.

Treatment

- As with supracondylar fractures, neurovascular assessment is needed.
- Undisplaced fractures may only require a backslab with the elbow flexed to 90°.
- Displaced fractures:
  - Likely to need complex surgery performed by a specialist surgeon.
  - Even then the elbow is likely to be stiff with decreased range of movement.
  - Osteoarthritis is not an uncommon late complication.

Complications

- Osteoarthritis
- Compartment syndrome
- Non-union
- Ulnar nerve palsy.

MICRO-print

Volkmann's ischaemic contracture is the permanent flexion contracture of the hand at the wrist following a period of ischaemia. This ischaemia can occur as a result of occlusion of the arterial supply to the arm. This may be due to damage to the brachial artery following a supracondylar fracture. Compartment syndrome can also occur after supra-condylar fractures due to swelling of the anterior compartment in the forearm. If untreated, ischaemic contracture can result.

MEDIAL EPICONDYLAR FRACTURES

- This may occur due to direct trauma or as a result of a valgus force being applied which results in an avulsion fracture. This can occur during dislocation of the elbow.
- The ulnar nerve is at risk of damage as it runs close to the medical epicondyle and therefore neurological status must be checked.

LATERAL EPICONDYLE AND CONDYLE FRACTURES

Again, these are often as a result of avulsion forces following a varus strain. They most commonly occur in children under the age of 10 years.

OLECRANON FRACTURES

There are two main mechanisms for fractures of the olecranon:
- A fall directly onto the flexed elbow or a direct blow to the elbow can result in a comminuted fracture.
- A fall onto the outstretched hand while the triceps muscle contracts may result in an avulsion fracture of the olecranon.

Treatment
- Undisplaced fractures may be treated closed with immobilization with a cast.
- Surgery, using tension band wiring or a plate, is recommended for displaced fractures of the olecranon.

Upper limb

6 Hand and wrist

6.1 OVERVIEW

For an overview of the anatomy of the hand and wrist, including dermatomes of the hand and peripheral nerve innervations, see Figs 6.1, 6.2 and 6.3.

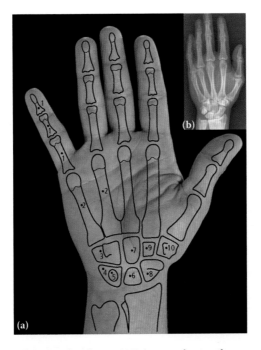

Fig. 6.1 Anatomy of the hand and wrist (a) Palmar surface surface anatomy: 1, proximal, middle and distal phalanges; 2, metacarpals; 3, hamate; 4, triquetral; 5, pisiform; 6, lunate; 7, capitate; 8, scaphoid; 9, trapezoid; 10, trapezium. (b) X-ray, dorsopalmar view. (c) Bones and muscle attachments, palmar aspect. Reproduced with permission from Abrahams P, Craven J, Lumley J. The wrist and hand. In: *Illustrated Clinical Anatomy*. London: Hodder Arnold, 2011.

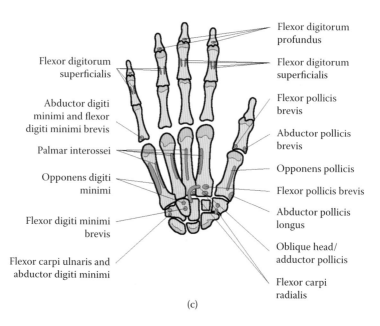

Flexor digitorum superficialis

Abductor digiti minimi and flexor digiti minimi brevis

Palmar interossei

Opponens digiti minimi

Flexor digiti minimi brevis

Flexor carpi ulnaris and abductor digiti minimi

Flexor digitorum profundus

Flexor digitorum superficialis

Flexor pollicis brevis

Abductor pollicis brevis

Opponens pollicis

Flexor pollicis brevis

Abductor pollicis longus

Oblique head/ adductor pollicis

Flexor carpi radialis

(c)

Fig. 6.1 (*Continued*)

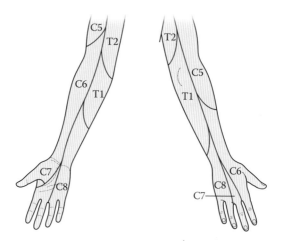

Fig. 6.2 Dermatomes of the hand. Medical illustration by Miss Alison Baxter.

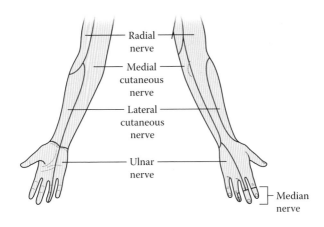

Fig. 6.3 Diagram of peripheral nerve innervations of hand (border of ulnar and median nerves). Medical illustration by Miss Alison Baxter.

HISTORY

Pathology of the hand or wrist can have a significant effect on activities of daily living. Enquire about specific loss of function.

Localize symptoms to the anatomical area. Establish the duration of symptoms and any precipitating factors. Ask about:

- Pain
- Stiffness
- Swelling
- Deformity

> **MICRO-facts**
>
> Remember adequate exposure of the arm is essential to fully assess a patient's hand and wrist.

EXAMINATION

Look

- Resting posture of the hand and wrist
- Scarring or discoloration
- Lumps or swellings (Table 6.1)

Table 6.1 Clinical signs which are found in hands.

DISEASE	WHAT TO LOOK FOR
Rheumatoid arthritis	Swan neck deformity, Boutonnière deformity, ulnar deviation of fingers, z-shaped thumb, radial deviation of the wrist, knuckle/wrist subluxation, rheumatoid nodules, swollen joints
Osteoarthritis	Bouchard's nodes, Heberden's nodes, squaring of the first carpometacarpal joint
Dupuytren's contracture	Fixed flexion of one or more fingers
Peripheral nerve injuries	Abnormal hand positions, muscle wasting (especially thenar and hypothenar muscles)
Gout	Gouty tophi
Ganglia	Swellings
Psoriasis	Plaques, nail pitting, onycholysis
Connective tissue disease	Splinter haemorrhages in the nails

Feel

- Temperature
- Any lumps should be examined for consistency and any attachment to overlying skin or underlying bone or tendon.
- Localize tenderness (Table 6.2).

Move

- Active and passive movements of each joint
- Grip strength
- Functional assessment, e.g. ask patient to hold a key, do up buttons, write with a pen.

Table 6.2 Important sites of tenderness in the hand and their relevant diagnoses.

SITE OF TENDERNESS	PROBABLE PATHOLOGY
Tip of the radial styloid	De Quervain's disease
Anatomical snuffbox	Scaphoid fracture
Base of the thumb	Carpometacarpal osteoarthritis
Generalized over wrist and finger joints	Rheumatoid arthritis or osteoarthritis
Ulnar side of the anatomical snuffbox	Tenosynovitis of extensor carpi radialis brevis
Distal end of ulna	Tenosynovitis of extensor carpi ulnaris

MICRO-facts

If the patient is also complaining of neck pain then a full neurological examination must also be carried out in case the wrist/hand pain is referred pain from problems such as cervical disc prolapse.

Pain could also be referred from a Pancoast tumour invading the brachial plexus so if suspected, perform a respiratory examination.

6.2 CARPAL TUNNEL SYNDROME

DEFINITION

Carpal tunnel syndrome is defined as compressive neuropathy of the median nerve at the wrist.

EPIDEMIOLOGY

- It is the most common compressive neuropathy.
- Female:male ratio of 3–5:1.
- Increased incidence in middle age.

AETIOLOGY

- Compression of the median nerve at the wrist due to hypertrophy of the flexor synovium.
- The causes of carpal tunnel syndrome can be remembered by the mnemonic ICRAMPS:
- ICRAMPS
  - **I**diopathic
  - **C**olles, Cushing's
  - **R**heumatoid
  - **A**cromegaly, amyloid
  - **M**yxoedema, mass, (diabetes) mellitus
  - **P**regnancy
  - **S**arcoid, systemic lupus erythromatosus (SLE).

MICRO-facts

The floor and walls of the carpal tunnel are bounded by the carpal bones. The flexor retinaculum creates the roof of the tunnel. The retinaculum attaches to the tubercle of the scaphoid and ridge of the trapezium radially, and the pisiform and the hook of the hamate on the ulnar side.

Upper limb

> **MICRO-case**
>
> Mrs Median is a 45-year-old secretary who presents to the orthopaedic clinic after several months of pain and pins and needles in her right hand. She says that the symptoms often come on in the middle of the night and she has to hang her hand over the bed for a few minutes to make them go away. She says that she could cope with the night symptoms, but now she is getting symptoms while she is typing at work which means she has to stop for a couple of minutes to make them go away. She is worried she will be sacked for not doing enough work.
>
> You make a diagnosis of carpal tunnel syndrome.
>
> **Points to consider**
> - Carpal tunnel syndrome often occurs in females in middle age.
> - Symptoms are brought on by the hands being in flexion, e.g. during typing, which reduces the carpal tunnel space, compresses the median nerve and causes symptoms.
> - Using wrist supports while typing may reduce symptoms as these will maintain a neutral position of the wrists.

PATHOPHYSIOLOGY

- Nerve fibres may be damaged by varying degrees.
- Neuropraxia is a reversible process where there is segmental demyelination of the nerve.
- With prolonged or severe compression, there may be axonal disruption. This is axonotmesis. Wasting of the thenar eminence occurs and is unlikely to recover.

> **MICRO-facts**
>
> Pain in carpal tunnel syndrome is thought to result from ischaemia rather than direct physical pressure on the nerve.

CLINICAL FEATURES

History

- Pain and paraesthesia in the thumb, index and middle fingers and radial half of the ring finger
- Symptoms often worse at night
- Dropping things
- Forearm pain.

EXAMINATION

- Hand may have normal appearance
- Weakness of thumb abduction
- Thenar wasting

- Tinel's sign: pain or paraesthesia on gentle tapping over the median nerve with the wrist in neutral
- Phalen's sign: passive flexion of wrist for up to 60 seconds provokes symptoms.

DIFFERENTIAL DIAGNOSIS

- Cervical radiculopathy
- Spinal cord lesion
- Peripheral neuropathy.

INVESTIGATIONS

- Nerve conduction studies

MANAGEMENT

- Conservative: Futura splint.
- Injection of steroid may provide short-term relief.
- Surgical carpal tunnel decompression.

6.3 ULNAR NERVE COMPRESSION

DEFINITION

- Compression of the ulnar nerve in the wrist or elbow.

EPIDEMIOLOGY

- Second most common compressive neuropathy.

AETIOLOGY

- Compression by: ganglia, malunion after fracture, prolonged flexion of the elbow
- Compression of the nerve can occur in Guyon's canal in the wrist or at the elbow in or around the cubital tunnel.

PATHOPHYSIOLOGY

- The pathophysiology is much the same as for carpal tunnel syndrome due to the mechanism of injury being the same.

CLINICAL FEATURES

History

- Pain and paraesthesia in the ulnar one and a half fingers
- Symptoms often worse at night.

EXAMINATION

- Clawing of the fingers
- Intrinsic muscle wasting

- Sensory loss over the ulnar nerve distribution
- Motor dysfunction
- Elbow flexion and tapping the ulnar nerve behind the medial epicondyle of the elbow causes symptoms and can help define the point of compression.

DIFFERENTIAL DIAGNOSIS

- Cervical radiculopathy
- Spinal cord lesion
- Peripheral neuropathy.

INVESTIGATIONS

- Nerve conduction studies

MANAGEMENT

- Conservative: wrist splints
- Surgical: decompression.

6.4 RADIAL NERVE LESIONS

DEFINITION

- Compression of the radial nerve

AETIOLOGY

- Often called 'Saturday night palsy' as the nerve is easily compressed in the axilla by falling asleep with an arm over a chair – a position sometimes adopted at the end of a night after too many drinks!
- Alternatively, the nerve may be damaged by humeral fractures, compression at the elbow, radial fractures, or compression by the extensor carpi radialis brevis.

PATHOPHYSIOLOGY

Pathophysiology is the same as for carpal tunnel syndrome.

CLINICAL FEATURES

History

- Pain distal to the elbow
- Weak wrists and fingers

EXAMINATION

- Wrist drop
- Weak metacarpophalangeal extension
- Sensory loss in the distribution of the radial nerve.

Upper limb

DIFFERENTIAL DIAGNOSIS

- Cervical radiculopathy
- Spinal cord lesion
- Peripheral neuropathy

INVESTIGATIONS

- Nerve conduction studies
- Ultrasound to help identify cause and site of lesion
- Magnetic resonance imaging (MRI) can help to identify the cause.

MANAGEMENT

- Conservative: wrist splints
- Surgical: exploration, tendon transfer, decompression.

6.5 DUPUYTREN'S DISEASE

DEFINITION

Contracture of the palmar fascia of the hand resulting in flexion deformities of the metacarpophalangeal (MCP) and the proximal interphalangeal (PIP) joints.

MICRO-facts

Ledderhose disease is contracture of the plantar fascia of the feet. This group of fibromatoses also includes penile fibromatosis (Peyronie disease) and fibromatosis of the dorsal PIP joints (Garrod nodes or knuckle pads).

EPIDEMIOLOGY

- Most patients with Dupuytren's disease are native to or descendants of ancestors from northern Europe.
- It is estimated that 4–6% of Caucasian populations have Dupuytren's disease.
- The disease is twice as common in men.

AETIOLOGY

- Genetic predisposition
- Other factors associated with the disease include:
  - Diabetes
  - Smoking
  - Liver disease.

PATHOPHYSIOLOGY

- The palmar fascia develops nodular, hypertrophic degeneration, adhering to the skin as it progresses. The dense fascia contracts, resulting in flexion deformity of the involved joints.
- Myofibroblasts are the predominant cell type.
- Normal fascia is primarily type I collagen, Dupuytren's disease is associated with increased type III collagen.

MICRO-facts

There are several hypotheses for the pathogenesis of Dupuytren's disease. Localized ischaemia results in free radical production with fibroblast proliferation and increased cytokine production. Fibroblasts differentiate to myofibroblasts and there is increased type III collagen deposition. The intrinsic theory states that the diseased tissue arises from existing fascia. The extrinsic theory suggests the Dupuytren's nodules arise *de novo* in the subdermal tissue and attaches to the overlying fascia.

CLINICAL FEATURES

History

- Thickening in the palm or digits
- Unable to fully straighten fingers
- Getting the hand caught on pocket
- The ring and little fingers are most commonly affected.

EXAMINATION

- Firm nodules, adherent to the skin
- Painless fibrous cords palpable in the palm
- Presence of MCP and PIP joint contractures.

MICRO-facts

Tabletop test of Hueston

Place the hand and fingers prone on a table. If positive, the hand will not go flat. A positive test may indicate surgery.

INVESTIGATIONS

- Dupuytren's disease is predominantly a clinical diagnoses.
- Ultrasound may demonstrate thickening of the fascia or be used to exclude differential diagnoses.

MANAGEMENT

- Mild disease can be managed conservatively.
- Fasciotomy involves simple division of Dupuytren's cords and may be done open or closed. Closed fasciotomy carries increased risk of neurovascular injury.
- Fasciectomy may be limited or extensive and involves excision of the diseased fascia.
- Occupational therapy with serial stretching and splinting is imperative post-operatively.
- Newer treatments include collagenase injection.

6.6 TENOSYNOVITIS

DEFINITION

Tenosynovitis is defined as synovial inflammation in a tendon sheath.

EPIDEMIOLOGY

- Often occurs during middle age
- Common in people who perform a repetitive movement each day, such as typing.

AETIOLOGY

- Trauma including repetitive wrist movements causing an inflammatory reaction of the tendon sheath
- Rheumatoid arthritis causing inflammation in tendon sheaths.

PATHOPHYSIOLOGY

Inflammation in a tendon sheath causes thickening and narrowing of the sheath, restricting the tendon within it.

CLINICAL FEATURES

The clinical features are dependent on the tendon affected.

History

- Pain along the length of a tendon, particularly on movement
- Restriction of movement.

EXAMINATION

- Swelling
- Tenderness
- Crepitus
- In De Quervain's disease, the tendon sheaths of the abductor pollicis longus and extensor pollicis brevis are involved, causing pain over the tip of the radial styloid.

Upper limb

- In trigger finger, the flexor tendon sheath in a finger or thumb is affected and a nodule can form on the sheath, preventing full extension. The nodule catches on movement causing the digit to 'snap' into flexion/extension.
- Golfer's elbow causes pain on the medial aspect of the elbow.
- Tennis elbow causes pain on the lateral aspect of the elbow.
- Achilles tendonitis causes pain above the heel in the Achilles tendon.

MICRO-facts

Finkelstein's test

Flexion of the thumb across the palm while adducting the wrist elicits pain in a positive test. Adducting the wrist without thumb flexion does not cause pain in de Quervain's disease.

INVESTIGATIONS

These are not usually indicated, but ultrasound or MRI can be performed if the diagnosis is unclear.

MANAGEMENT

- Conservative:
  - Rest
  - Wrist splints
  - Non-steroidal anti-inflammatory drugs (NSAIDs)
  - Steroid injections
- Surgical:
  - Tendon sheath decompression.

6.7 GANGLIA

- Fluid-filled cysts formed from synovium and filled with synovial fluid.
- Usually affect young adults, but not exclusively.
- Aetiology and pathophysiology is unknown.
- Commonly found around the wrist or on feet.
- Ganglia are usually painless, although they may sometimes cause discomfort. They typically fluctuate in size insidiously.
- On examination, they are hard, painless masses with a smooth outline which transluminate.
- Differentials depend on the site where they occur, but could include rheumatoid nodules, joint effusions, tumours, neurofibromas.
- Further investigations are not usually needed unless other pathology needs to be excluded, in which case x-rays, ultrasound scans and MRIs can be performed as necessary.

- Treatment is not necessary, but if desired, ganglia can be removed by aspiration or surgical excision, although recurrence is likely.

6.8 RHEUMATOID ARTHRITIS, OSTEOARTHRITIS, CRYSTAL ARTHROPATHIES

These conditions have been covered fully in other chapters and so the information will not be repeated here. Refer to the relevant chapters (see Chapter 11, Rheumatoid arthritis; Chapter 16, Non-inflammatory arthroses; and Chapter 15, Crystal arthropathies, for more about each of these diseases).

6.9 ENCHONDROMA

- These are relatively common benign primary bone tumours.
- Most common in young people but do not usually cause any symptoms.
- The tumour originates from pieces of cartilage left inside bones.
- Although often found in the hand, they can be present in other areas such as the feet and long bones.
- These tumours do not normally cause any symptoms, although they may cause a lump and rarely pain.
- X-ray is the optimal imaging modality to diagnose these lesions.
- Treatment is not usually needed unless the tumour is growing, causing pain or swelling, or if it manifests as a fracture. In the above cases, the tumour is removed by curettage.
- Note. There is a very small risk of malignant change in these tumours.

6.10 MALLET FINGER

- An injury commonly sustained when trying to catch a ball.
- Common in sports players, such as cricketers.
- The method of injury is that the terminal phalanx is suddenly pushed into hyper-flexion, rupturing the extensor tendon.
- On examination, the terminal phalanx will appear dropped and the patient is unable to actively extend the terminal phalanx at the distal interphalangeal joint. There may be accompanying swelling.
- Treatment can either be by conservative management with finger splinting, or surgical intervention by inserting Kirschner wires.

6.11 DISTAL RADIAL FRACTURES

AETIOLOGY

- Often eponymously named as a Colles' (dorsal displacement) or Smith's fracture (volar displacement).
- Colles' fractures are often also angulated radially.

Upper limb

- If there is accompanying radio-carpal dislocation, it is called a Barton's fracture
- Common in patients with osteoporosis, typically postmenopausal women.

MECHANISM OF INJURY

- **Colles' fracture** is usually the result of a person falling with their arms stretched out in front of them which means the distal part of the radius is pushed dorsally on impact with the floor.
- **Smith's fracture** occurs after falling on a flexed wrist which means the distal part of the radius is pushed in a volar direction on impact.
- **Barton's fracture** is dorsal or volar distal radial displacement, but with accompanying radio-carpal dislocation. The mechanism of injury is usually the same as for Colles' or Smith's fractures.

ANATOMICAL CONSIDERATIONS

- It is important to check there is no median/ulnar nerve damage.
- In Barton's fractures particularly, tendons and blood vessels can get trapped.

ASSESSMENT

- Colles': a classic 'dinner fork' deformity is seen (Fig. 6.4).
- Smith's: a 'garden spade' deformity occurs (Fig. 6.4).
- Always check neurovascular status of the limb.
- X-rays: PA and lateral views.

(a)

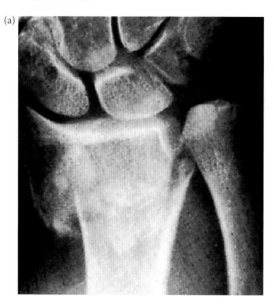

Fig. 6.4 (a,b) Colles' fracture. (c,d) Smith's fracture. Reproduced with permission from Solomon L, Warwick D, Nayagam S (eds.). *Apley's Concise Orthopaedics and Fractures*, 9th edn. London: Hodder Arnold, 2010.

(b)

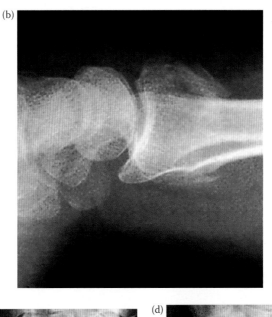

(c)

(d)

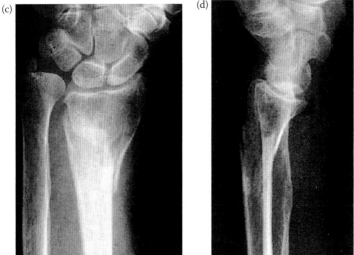

Fig. 6.4 (*Continued*)

MANAGEMENT

- Colles' fracture:
    - Conservative – reduction (under anaesthetic) followed by immobilisation in a cast.
    - Surgical – Usually for more complex cases and the type of surgery depends on the individual case.
- Smith's:
    - Often these are unstable and so treatment is usually surgical (open reduction and internal fixation).

Note. Colles' and Smith's fractures are extra-articular fractures. Intra-articular distal radial fractures lead to dorsal and volar subluxation of the wrist and hence instability.

Internal fixation is needed to reduce the chance of secondary osteoarthritis.

6.12 SCAPHOID FRACTURES

DEFINITION

- The scaphoid is the most commonly fractured carpal bone.
- It is more common for a young person to sustain a scaphoid fracture than a distal radial fracture, even though the mechanism of injury is often the same.

MECHANISM OF INJURY

- These are usually sustained after falling onto an outstretched hand.

ANATOMICAL CONSIDERATIONS

- The important point to remember about scaphoid fractures is that they are prone to non-union and avascular necrosis. This is because the blood supply enters at the distal portion of the bone through the nutrient artery, so the more proximal the fracture the higher the risk of this happening.

ASSESSMENT

- Classically, there is pain on palpation of the anatomical snuffbox and/or on the scaphoid tuberosity, as well as on wrist movements.
- X-rays: anteroposterior, lateral and oblique views.
- Note. It is often hard to spot these fractures on x-ray immediately after the injury and may only become apparent on subsequent follow up x-rays.
- If a fracture is highly suspected but not visible on x-rays, other imaging modalities such as bone scintillation, MRI and CT may be used.

MANAGEMENT

Immediate treatment is dependent on whether the fracture is displaced or not:
- **Undisplaced**: immobilization in a cast, for how long depends on the exact site of injury but ranges from 6 to 24 weeks
- **Displaced**: surgery (open reduction and internal fixation).

6.13 CONGENITAL DEFORMITIES

- You should be aware that congenital deformities of the hand are very common.
- Although you do not need to know the details of these congenital deformities as an undergraduate, you should be aware of them.
- They include:
  - Failure of formation of the fingers or hand (transverse failure)
  - Failure of formation of the central aspect, radial or ulnar side of the arm and hand (longitudinal failure)
  - Webbing of the fingers (syndactyly)
  - Extra digits (polydactyly)
  - Big digits (macrodactyly)
  - Constriction bands formed around the hand or fingers
- Note that the presence of some of these may indicate congenital abnormalities of other organs.
- Syndromes affecting multiple areas of the body, such as arthrogryposis, can also affect the hand.
- Syndromes such as Down syndrome can have characteristic features in the hand, e.g. a short 5th finger.

Upper limb

Sacrum and pelvis

7.1 OVERVIEW

The sacrum and pelvis are areas often overlooked by medical students when learning about orthopaedics.

This chapter will concentrate on the individual pathologies and trauma affecting the sacrum and pelvis, as opposed to the history and examination.

7.2 ANATOMY OF THE SACRUM AND PELVIS

The anatomy of the pelvis is shown in Fig. 7.1. The bony pelvis is made up of the sacrum and three fused bones bilaterally:

- Ilium
- Pubis
- Ischium.

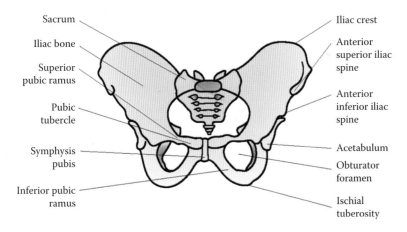

Fig. 7.1 Anatomy of the pelvis. Reproduced with permission from Abrahams P, Craven J, Lumley J. The upper limb. In: *Illustrated Clinical Anatomy*. London: Hodder Arnold, 2011.

The three fused bones on each side are connected to the sacrum by the sacroiliac ligaments posteriorly. Anteriorly, the two sides of the pelvis are joined together by the pubic symphysis, which means it forms the shape of a ring. The function of the pelvis is to protect internal structures and aid in transferring weight from the spine to the legs.

MICRO-facts

The pelvis differs in structure in males and females as the female pelvis is designed to accommodate the processes of childbirth. Such differences include a heart-shaped pelvic inlet in men, whereas in women it is more of an oval shape.

7.3 ANKYLOSING SPONDYLITIS

This condition is one of the spondyloarthropathies and so is discussed in more detail in Chapter 13, Spondyloarthritides. However, it has important manifestations in the sacral and pelvic regions.

- An early sign of the disease is pain and tenderness of the sacroiliac joints with corresponding abnormalities on x-ray over this area, including destruction and sclerosis.
- As the disease progresses, fusion of the joint can occur.
- Treatment includes physiotherapy, non-steroidal anti-inflammatory drugs (NSAIDs), or hip replacement, as the hips are commonly affected.

7.4 OSTEOMALACIA

- Osteomalacia is discussed further in Chapter 17, Disorders of bone metabolism. Please refer to this section for more information.
- This is a disease where osteoid fails to be mineralized. It can be due to various abnormalities such as vitamin D malabsorption, malnutrition or Fanconi syndrome.
- Characteristically, there are fractures and Looser's zones on x-ray of the pelvis with corresponding pain.
- Treatment is with vitamin D.

MICRO-facts

Looser's zones denote where there is translucency in the bone. They are found in osteomalacia.

7.5 TUBERCULOSIS

Tuberculosis may be a cause of gradual onset pain. It is covered in greater detail in Chapter 3, Thoracic and lumbar spine.

7.6 NEOPLASTIC PATHOLOGY

While it is unnecessary to know about pelvic and sacral neoplastic pathology in detail as an undergraduate, for completeness, here are some which are commonly associated with this region:

- **Benign:** commonly chondromas and osteochondromas
- **Malignant:** chondrosarcoma, multiple myeloma and metastases from other sites of malignancy in the body.

7.7 SACRAL INJURIES

MECHANISM OF INJURY

Often, sacral injuries result from falling directly on to a hard surface causing a blow to the sacrum.

ANATOMICAL CONSIDERATIONS

Injuries to the sacrum can involve the sacral nerves

ASSESSMENT

Due to the possible involvement of the sacral nerves, it should be checked to see whether the patient has corresponding symptoms such as:

- Loss of sensation
- Incontinence
- Leg weakness

X-rays of the pelvic inlet and pelvic outlet (true anteroposterior (AP)) should be undertaken.

MANAGEMENT

- These fractures rarely need surgery unless there are persistent neurological symptoms or the urinary tract has been disturbed.
- If a fracture is displaced, reduction might be indicated.
- Advise the use of a rubber ring cushion when sitting to aid the patient's comfort.

7.8 PELVIC INJURIES

MECHANISM OF INJURY

- Often these are the result of major trauma, such as a road traffic accident.
- In these cases, it is paramount that the patient is properly assessed, as resuscitation may need to be attempted first. Follow Advanced Trauma Life Support (ATLS) guidelines.

Upper limb

ANATOMICAL CONSIDERATIONS

- Due to the proximity of parts of the urinary tract, bowel, major blood vessels and nerves to the pelvic bones, damage to these structures is possible after pelvic fracture.
- Remember: a large amount of blood can collect in the pelvis causing the patient to become shocked which can be life threatening.
- The ambulance crew will have put a pelvic binder on a patient who is suspected to have a pelvic ring fracture to minimize internal bleeding.
- Alternatively, a bed sheet can be tied around the pelvis to produce the same effect.

ASSESSMENT

- The type of imaging that can be done depends on the stability of the patient.
- At a minimum, an anteroposterior (AP) x-ray of the pelvis should be performed.
- Computed tomography (CT) scan should be performed if the patient is stable and it is indicated.
- Intravenous urogram should be performed if damage to the urinary tract is suspected.

MICRO-facts

Urethral injury

Urethral injury should be suspected when:
- The prostate is high riding on digital rectal examination.
- There is blood at the meatus and the patient is unable to pass urine (this would also occur if the bladder has ruptured).

MANAGEMENT

Stable fractures

- Avulsion fractures. These occur when a muscle contracts and pulls off a piece of bone to which it is attached during the process.
- An example of a site where this occurs in the pelvis is the rectus femoris pulling on the anterior inferior iliac spine.
- Most of these fractures just need rest and symptomatic relief, but depending on the site and severity, open reduction and internal fixation may be necessary.

Single fractures

These are usually caused by direct force on the bone and include sites such as:

- Superior pubic rami
- Sacrum extending into the sacroiliac joint
- Iliac wing, among other sites.

Once injury to the renal tract has been excluded, treatment should include rest, early mobilization and symptom relief.

Complex fractures

- These can be stable or unstable depending on their severity and classification.
- There are three main directions of compression in these injuries, which include anteroposterior, lateral and vertical forces.
- Anteroposterior compression:
  - Causes what is known as an 'open book' fracture. These may involve the symphysis pubis, pubic rami, sacroiliac joints and ileum.
  - Major blood loss is commonly associated with these fractures.
  - Treatment depends on the severity of the fracture and ranges from rest to fixation.
- Lateral compression:
  - Results in fractures of the pubic rami, ilium, sacrum or sacroiliac joint.
  - Like open book fractures, the treatment of these fractures depends on the exact injury and severity; therefore treatment ranges from rest to fixation.
- Vertical compression:
  - Causes the pubic rami to fracture, as well as the sacroiliac joint, sacrum or ileum on the same side.
  - Haemorrhage and sacral plexus nerve damage is commonly associated with these injuries.
  - Treatment includes reduction by either fixation or traction.

Note. Some injuries are a mixture of the above three patterns.

Acetabular fractures

- An example of an acetabular fracture is when the knees hit the dashboard in a road traffic accident and the subsequent force is transmitted up the femur, through the femoral head and causes a fracture of the acetabulum.
- The anterior and posterior columns and acetabular floor all need to be assessed in these cases. This will involve specialized x-rays or computed tomography (CT) scans.
- Treatment depends on the exact injury, but can include traction, physiotherapy, open reduction and internal fixation.
- Complications of these fractures include osteoarthritis.

Upper limb

MICRO-case

Ian Jury is a 45-year-old teacher who was knocked off his bike by a car while cycling to school 30 minutes ago. You are the junior doctor on-call for orthopaedics and are bleeped to come to the resuscitation unit in the Emergency Department when the air ambulance crew brings him in. They tell you he was hit side-on by a car travelling at 50 mph and was thrown a long distance from his bike. He has extensive injuries and has a Glasgow Coma Score (GCS) of 3/15.

Points to consider

- This man has been involved in a major trauma accident.
- He needs to be managed using the airway, breathing, circulation, disability, exposure (ABCDE) approach and resuscitated. Advanced Trauma Life Support (ATLS) guidelines need to be followed.
- If you suspect this man has had a pelvic injury, a pelvic binder needs to be put on, or at the very least a bed sheet tied tightly around the pelvis.

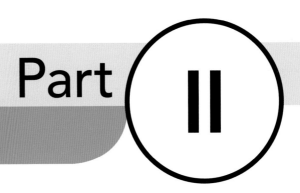

Lower limb

8 Hip

8.1 HIP OVERVIEW

The hip joint is a ball and socket synovial joint between the acetabulum and the head of femur (Fig. 8.1).

The hip joint requires two qualities: mobility and stability

MOBILITY

The hip propels the body in locomotion. This is made possible by a long and angled neck of femur together with a smooth articular cartilage which decreases friction during hip movement.

STABILITY

The hip supports major dynamic forces. It has a thick, fibrous capsule with strong hip ligaments which comprise:
- Iliofemoral – anterior
- Pubofemoral – medial
- Ischiofemoral – posterior
- Intracapsular – head of femur.

TAKING A 'HIP HISTORY' (A BRIEF REMINDER OF HOW TO TAKE A MUSCULOSKELETAL HISTORY)

A systematic approach
- Presenting complaint – remember 'hip pain is groin pain'
- Hip pathology can present with knee pain, especially in children, beware!
- History of presenting complaint
- SOCRATES (site, onset, character, radiation, associated findings, timing, exacerbating/relieving factors, severity)
- Impact of problem (social, domestic, work)
- Past medical history
- Family history, including congenital hip problems
- Drug history
- Social history (including occupation)

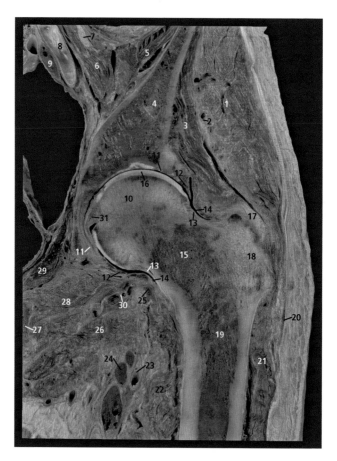

Fig. 8.1 Anatomy of the hip. 1, Gluteus medius; 2, superior gluteal neurovascular bundle; 3, gluteus minimus; 4, ilium; 5, iliacus; 6, psoas major; 7, femoral nerve; 8, external iliac artery; 9, external iliac vein; 10, head of femur; 11, rim of acetabulum; 12, acetabular labrum; 13, zona orbicularis of capsule; 14, capsule of hip joint; 15, neck of femur; 16, articular cartilage; 17, iliofemoral ligament; 18, greater trochanter; 19, shaft of femur; 20, iliotibial tract; 21, vastus lateralis; 22, vastus medialis; 23, profunda femoris artery; 24, profunda femoris vein; 25, iliopsoas tendon; 26, adductor longus; 27, ischiopubic ramus; 28, obturator externus; 29, obturator internus; 30, medial circumflex femoral artery and vein; 31, ligament of head of femur (ligamentum teres). Reproduced with permission from Ellis H, Logan BM, Dixon A. *Human Sectional Anatomy: Atlas of Body Sections, CT and MRI Images*, 3rd edn. London: Hodder Arnold, 2008.

- Systems enquiry: note that knee pain can be the only complaint of hip pathology and could be missed if you are not thorough.

MICRO-facts

Reminder of general examination principles:
- Explain to the patient beforehand what you are doing.
- Do not cause any undue pain or discomfort.
- Compare sides.
- Also examine joints above and below (i.e. spine and knee).

HIP EXAMINATION

- With the patient standing
  - Inspect the front, side and back of the patient with the hips exposed.
  - Perform the Trendelenburg's test to assess hip stability.
  - Ask the patient to walk several feet, turn and walk back to the starting position.
- With the patient supine
  - Inspection 1: Symmetry. Are the Anterior Superior Iliac Spines (ASIS) and the medial malleoli at the same levels?
  - Inspection 2: Abnormal hip contour(s), loss of muscle bulk, scars (+ asymmetrical skin creases in babies)
  - Lower limb measurement
  - As above, ensure the pelvis is straight with the ASIS at the same level.
  - With a measuring tape measure the length from the ASIS to the medial malleoli of each leg = 'Real' leg length
  - 'Apparent' length may be different to true length if there is a fixed deformity present, such as a tilted pelvis or flexion deformity of the hip. This is confirmed using Thomas' test (see Table 8.1).
  - Palpation
  - Never forget temperature! Use the back of your hand (a useful indicator for an inflammatory joint pathology).
  - Feel for the greater trochanters. Tenderness may be elicited.

MICRO-facts

Trendelenburg test

- With patient standing unassisted, ask them to lift one foot and flex at the knee (not the hip).
- Trendelenburg +ve (i.e. unstable hip): the pelvis drops to the unsupported side.
- Causes of +ve: Hip pain, hip abductor weakness, shortened femoral neck and dislocation, subluxation, disease of the femoral head.

continued...

Lower limb

continued...

- Surface marking of the femoral head is halfway between the ASIS and the pubic tubercle.
- This is also the surface marking of the deep inguinal ring.
- Movement
  - Pelvic tilt can compensate for leg shortening. Thomas' test is used to 'obliterate' pelvic tilt by neutralizing compensatory lumbar lordosis.
  - Thomas' test involves flexing both hips then extending one hip gently. If there is a fixed flexion deformity, the posterior aspect of the knee of the extended leg cannot touch the couch.
  - Abduction. Again, the pelvis needs to be fixed, but this time in the coronal plane. To do this, hang the other leg over the couch in full abduction before moving the leg to be examined.
  - Adduction. Cross the legs. Full adduction occurs when the pelvis begins to tilt.
  - Active range of movement. Elicit full joint range in the patient.
  - Ask patient to perform the following movements and note range (normal range in brackets):
    - Abduct (0–45°)
    - Adduct (0–30°)
    - Flexion (0–140°)
    - Internal rotation in hip flexion (0–40°)
    - External rotation in hip flexion (0–50°)
    - Extension with patient lying on their side (0–10°)
    - Repeat movements passively (feel the joint for crepitus) (Fig. 8.2)

Table 8.1 **Summary of special tests.**

TEST	HOW	POSITIVE SIGN	CAUSES
Trendelenburg	Stand: flex one hip	Pelvis tilts down to unsupported side	Pain or femoral head pathology, shortened femoral neck, weak abductors
Thomas'	Flex both hips: lower one leg	Posterior aspect of knee of leg lowered unable to touch couch	Fixed flexion deformity of the hip due to hip disease

ABDUCTION NOT A SPECIFIC TEST

A useful clue in diagnosing hip pathology is the age of the patient. Table 8.2 is a chronological table of conditions at different life stages.

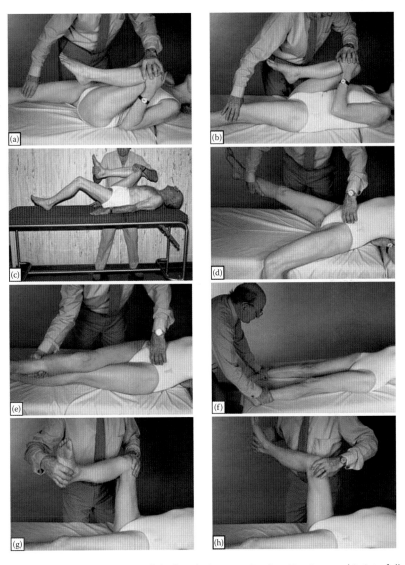

Fig. 8.2 Passive movements of the hip during examination. Forcing one hip into full flexion will straighten out the lumbar spine; the other hip should still be capable of full extension in this position. (b) Now the position is reversed; the right hip is held in full flexion. (c) If the hip cannot straighten out completely, this is referred to as a *fixed flexion deformity*. (d) Testing for abduction. The pelvis is kept level by placing the opposite leg over the edge of the examination couch with that hip also in abduction (the examiner's left hand checks the position of the anterior spines) before abducting the target hip. (e) Testing for adduction. (f–h) External and internal rotation are assessed (f) first with the hips in full extension and then (g, h) in 90 degrees of flexion. (i) Testing for extension. Reproduced with permission from Solomon L, Warwick D, Nayagam S. *Apley's Concise System Orthopaedics and Fractures*, 3rd edn. London: Hodder Arnold, 2005.

Lower limb

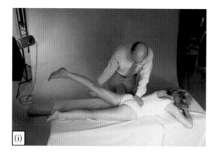

(i)

Fig. 8.2 (*Continued*)

Table 8.2 **Age versus hip pathology.**

AGE (YEARS)	PROBABLE HIP PATHOLOGY
Newborn	Developmental dysplasia of the hip (DDH)
0–5	Infection/late presentation of DDH
4–9	Perthes' disease
11–17	Slipped upper femoral epiphysis (SUFE)
Adult	Osteoarthritis/rheumatoid Arthritis

Adapted from Solomon L, Warwick D, Nayagam S. *Apley's Concise System of Orthopaedics and Fractures*, 3rd edn. London: Hodder Arnold, 2005.

8.2 DEVELOPMENTAL DYSPLASIA OF THE HIP

DEFINITION

Includes a range of congenital hip instabilities varying from shallow acetabulum to frank dislocation with the femoral head slipping outside the acetabulum.

EPIDEMIOLOGY

Between 1 and 2% of neonates are affected. Girls are affected seven times more than boys.

AETIOLOGY

Risk factors are family history and breech delivery.

INVESTIGATIONS

Tests

Click test of Otolani and Barlow's manoeuvre. Ideally, all neonates should be screened. At 6 weeks, ultrasound may be used.

MANAGEMENT

Reduce hips

- Double nappies
- Abduction splint (Parlik harness) for the first three to six months.
- Late presentation (>18 months) may require open reduction.
- Surgery is usually used to reduce a dislocated hip. If left untreated, it leads to hip deformity and disability.

MICRO-facts

Click test of Ortolani

In supine position, flex the hips and slowly abduct one hip in turn. Positive Ortolani is demonstrated by a palpable and often audible click as the head of femur slips back into the shallow acetabulum indicating hip instability.

MICRO-facts

Barlow's manoeuvre

Stabilize the pelvis with one hand and with other hand abduct each hip to 45°. Pressing with the thumb into the groin will lead to the femoral head slipping out of the acetabulum if the hip is unstable (positive test).

Note: Avoid repetition of these tests as they may aggravate hip instability.

8.3 HIP INFECTION

Hip infections need to be diagnosed early and treated aggressively.

AETIOLOGY

Organism usually staphylococcus from local femoral osteomyelitis or blood-borne distant foci.

CLINICAL FEATURES

Child may be septic and if so will resist attempts to move hip (pseudo-paralysis).

INVESTIGATIONS

X-ray may show joint displacement secondary to effusion. Joint aspirate should be taken for micro-investigation.

Lower limb

MANAGEMENT

Antibiotics should be given, both intravenously and into the joint. Splinting the hip is advisable until infection has resolved.

Note: Tuberculosis should be in your differential diagnosis if the patient is in an at-risk group.

8.4 PERTHES' DISEASE

DEFINITION

Perthes' disease is necrosis of the femoral head.

EPIDEMIOLOGY

It is rare and usually occurs in 4–9 year olds.

AETIOLOGY

Perthes' disease is caused by developmental changes in the blood supply to the femoral head making the femoral head susceptible to necrosis.

CLINICAL FEATURES

Clinically, the child will have a limp with limited abduction and internal rotation.

INVESTIGATION

X-ray should be taken to detect increased joint space and increased density of epiphysis.

MANAGEMENT

Treatment is by splinting the hip. Severe cases may require osteotomy.

MICRO-print
Blood supply to femoral head at 4-7 years old

Before the age of four years, the femoral head is supplied by the metaphyseal vessels, lateral epiphyseal vessels in the retinaculum and developing vessels in the ligamentum teres. Between four and seven years, the femoral head may only depend on the lateral supply, which is vulnerable to stretch if there is a hip effusion.

8.5 SLIPPED UPPER FEMORAL EPIPHYSIS

DEFINITION

Slipped upper femoral epiphysis (SUFE) is defined by displacement of the epiphyseal growth plate.

EPIDEMIOLOGY

It mainly affects overweight pubescent boys.

CLINICAL FEATURES

Clinical presentation is with sudden onset groin, hip or referred knee pain, potentially secondary to trauma. The leg is shortened and externally rotated.

INVESTIGATIONS

Investigation is by x-ray to detect a widened epiphyseal plate.

MANAGEMENT

Management is by epiphyseal pinning and osteotomy in severe cases.

8.6 OSTEOARTHRITIS

Both osteoarthritis (OA) and rheumatoid arthritis (RA) are addressed in more detail later in the book (see Chapter 11, Rheumatoid arthritis and Chapter 16, Non-inflammatory arthroses).

Hip osteoarthritis is very common in older adults (>50 years).

AETIOLOGY

It is usually idiopathic, but may be secondary to Perthe's, rheumatoid arthritis, Paget's or avascular necrosis (AVN).

CLINICAL FEATURES

It presents with progressive groin pain after sustained movement ('end of the day'). Examination can reveal positive Trendelenburg and Thomas' tests.

INVESTIGATION

Investigation is by x-ray to detect loss of joint space, osteophytes, sclerosis and subchrondral cysts (LOSS).

MANAGEMENT

Management is by physiotherapy, non-steroidal anti-inflammatory drugs (NSAIDs), hip arthoplasty or total hip replacement.

8.7 RHEUMATOID ARTHRITIS

DEFINITION

Rheumatoid arthritis is classically a small joint polyarthropathy. Usually the patient will already have other joints affected by RA.

Lower limb

CLINICAL FEATURES

Clinical features include progressive joint destruction with early morning pain which improves with joint movement (as opposed to OA). On examination, restricted movement and muscle wasting may be evident.

INVESTIGATIONS

Investigations include x-ray to detect osteoporosis, joint erosion and destruction.

MANAGEMENT

Treatment involves NSAIDs, corticosteroids, biological agents (see Chapter 11, Rheumatoid arthritis for drug groups) and total hip replacement.

8.8 FRACTURE OF NECK OF FEMUR

EPIDEMIOLOGY

Fractures occur in all age groups. Older females are particularly susceptible due to post-menopausal osteoporosis.

RISK FACTORS

Risk factors are female gender, age, osteoporosis, 'frequent faller' (many causes such as poor eyesight, medications, cardiac conditions, postural hypotension, Parkinson's disease and dementia, for example).

CLINICAL PRESENTATION

- Shortening and external rotation of hip.
- X-ray: loss of length of femoral neck
- Sites: Intra or extracapsular fracture
- Garden classification is commonly used to describe intra-capsular femoral neck fractures:
    - I. Stable with impaction
    - II. Complete but no displacement
    - III. Displaced with contact between fragments
    - IV. Displaced with no contact between fragments.
- The basic distinction between non-displaced (I–II) and displaced (III–IV) fractures is clinically significant as complication rates are much higher with grades III–IV.
- Intracapsular complication: femoral head ischaemia (known as avascular necrosis (AVN) of the femoral head). This is due to the main arterial supply to the head of the femur being compromised.
- The blood supply to the femoral head runs in the posterior capsule which can be torn in displaced fractures.

MANAGEMENT

- Dynamic hip screw (extracapsular).
- Hemiarthroplasty or total hip replacement for displaced intracapsular fractures.
- *In situ* pinning for undisplaced intracapsular fractures.
- Externally rotated and shortened leg?
- Shortening and external rotation of the hip is due to the excessive pull of the psoas muscle, which effectively pulls the leg up and outwards.

9 Knee

9.1 KNEE OVERVIEW

The knee is a modified synovial hinge joint. It is formed from the distal femur, the patella and the tibial plateau (Fig. 9.1). The bony structures do not provide much inherent stability and so most of the joint's stability comes from the surrounding ligaments, tendons and muscle action.

KNEE EXAMINATION

Inspection

- Ensure both legs are fully exposed.
- Ask the patient to walk and then to stand facing you, side on and away from you. This may provide early clues as to what is wrong with the patient. Any varus or valgus deformity should be noted along with assessment of muscle bulk, especially the quadriceps. Swellings and scars may be observed.
- With the patient lying down, view the patient from the end of the couch. Look for:
  - Swelling
  - Redness
  - Deformity
  - Rashes
  - Scars
  - Wasting of the muscles (particularly the vastus medialis).

Palpation

- Using the back of your hand, compare the temperature of each knee joint.
- With the legs still in relaxed extension, palpate along the joint line including around the patella. Do this while looking at the patient's face for any signs of discomfort.
  - With the knee flexed to 90°, palpate the joint line. With your fingers gently gripping behind the knee, using your thumbs beginning at the tibial tuberosity, methodically work your way around the joint to include the patella tendon, borders of the patella, and medial and lateral femoral and tibial condyles.

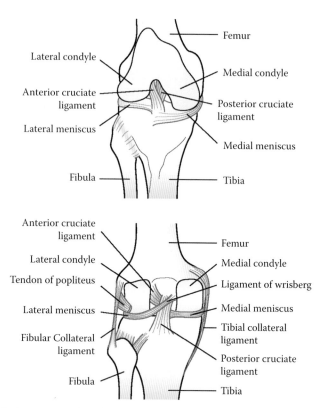

Fig. 9.1 Basic anatomy of the knee. Reproduced with permission from Williams N, Bulstrode C, O'Connell R. *Bailey & Love's Short Practice of Surgery*, 26th edn. London: Hodder Arnold, 2013.

- Feel for swelling of the joint by performing the patella tap test or fluid bulge sweep (Fig. 9.2).

Movement

- Starting with active movement, elicit full joint range in the patient. Ask patient to perform the following movements and note range.
  - Knee extension (0°)
  - Knee flexion: ask the patient to bring their heel to their buttock (150°).
- Repeat these movements passively with one hand placed over the patella, noting any crepitus.

9.2 SPECIAL TESTS IN THE KNEE

There are several special tests for the knee joint to assess the stability of the ligaments.

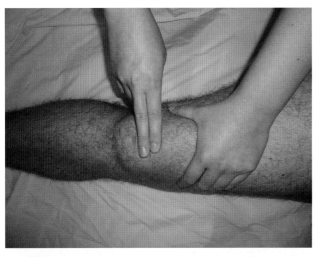

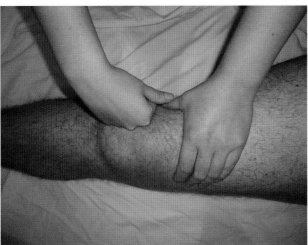

Fig. 9.2 The patella tap test or fluid bulge sweep.

ANTERIOR CRUCIATE LIGAMENT

Lachman test

With the knee in 20° of flexion, use one hand to grip the lower thigh and the other to grip the upper calf. The two hands can then be moved in opposite directions back and forth to assess the degree of laxity. Note: this test is more sensitive than the anterior draw test, however, it is more difficult if you have small hands or the patient has large legs.

Lower limb

Anterior drawer test

- With the patient's knee flexed to 90°, grip the lower leg from either side so that thumbs are placed over the tibial tuberosity and the fingers are placed behind the knee ensuring that the hamstrings are relaxed.
- Support the lower leg with your forearm and slowly draw forwards.
- If there is a deficiency in the anterior cruciate ligament (ACL), then there will be significant forward movement felt.
- As a slight amount of movement is normal, comparison of both sides can be helpful in identifying any abnormality (provided the contralateral side is normal).

POSTERIOR CRUCIATE LIGAMENT

Posterior sag

With the patient's knees flexed to 90° and the thighs resting on a pillow, look carefully from the side and compare. A deficit in the posterior cruciate ligament (PCL) may result in a visible step as the tibia sags backwards.

MEDIAL AND LATERAL COLLATERAL LIGAMENTS

- With the patient's knee in 20° of flexion, grip the heel and with the other hand on the medial aspect of the knee, apply a varus strain.
- Compare both sides and any significant difference suggests a lateral collateral ligament injury.
- Repeat this process, but this time use your hand on the lateral aspect of the knee to provide a valgus strain to assess the function of the medial collateral ligament.

MENISCUS

McMurray's test

- Flex the patient's hip to 90° and fully flex the patient's knee.
- With one hand on the heel of the foot and the other hand over the patella, externally rotate the knee and slowly extend the leg.
- Repeat the test, but with internal rotation of the knee and compare both sides.
- If this test results in a painful, audible, palpable click, then this suggests damage to the meniscus. Types of meniscal tear are discussed below under Meniscal injury.
- For completeness when examining the knee, the neurovascular status should also be examined and the hip and ankle should also be fully checked for problems.
- Beware! Knee pain may actually be referred pain from the hip.

9.3 COMMON KNEE PATHOLOGY

OSTEOARTHRITIS

- Although covered in greater detail in Chapter 16, Non-inflammatory arthroses, it is important to highlight osteoarthritis in this chapter as the knee is one of the most commonly affected joints.
- The osteoarthritis may be secondary to trauma, ligament damage, deformity or infection, but may also occur without any apparent cause.
- The most common presenting feature is pain, which initially may be related to activity, but may be present all the time as the osteoarthritis progresses.
- The medial compartment is more commonly affected, resulting in a varus deformity.
- Crepitus is often felt throughout flexion and extension of the knee.
- X-rays (Fig. 9.3) of the joint show a typical appearance of:
  - Loss of joint space
  - Osteophytes
  - Subchondral cysts
  - Subchondral sclerosis.
- Treatment initially is conservative, but as symptoms worsen, arthroplasty must be considered.
  - The aims of the knee replacement surgery are to reduce pain and correct any deformity.
  - Outcomes are excellent for this operation.

(a) 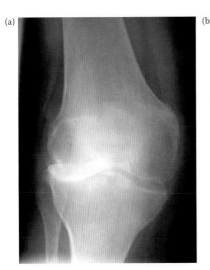 (b)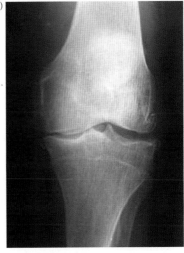

Fig. 9.3 X-ray of the knee showing osteoarthritic changes (a) and (b). Reproduced with permission from Williams N, Bulstrode C, O'Connell R. *Bailey & Love's Short Practice of Surgery*, 26th edn. London: Hodder Arnold, 2013.

Lower limb

RHEUMATOID ARTHRITIS

Rheumatoid arthritis (RA) is covered in Chapter 11, Rheumatoid arthritis. It may occasionally start in the knee, but typically other joints will be involved.

- The knee may be swollen and warm to the touch.
- There is muscle wasting, synovial thickening, tenderness and pain.
- A valgus deformity is more commonly seen in patients with RA.

OSTEOCHONDRITIS DISSECANS

Definition

This is damage to the maturing epiphysis. It can occur at any joint, but usually affects the knee.

Epidemiology

- Affects teenagers and those in their early twenties
- More common in males.
- Affects the femoral condyle, most commonly the lateral aspect of the medial condyle.

Aetiology

- Occurs when a segment of bone and overlying cartilage separates from the femoral condyle after undergoing avascular necrosis.
- This can result in the formation of a loose body within the joint.
- The most likely cause is trauma.
- Steroids are a risk factor.

Clinical features

Patients are likely to present with vague symptoms of an aching joint that swells after activity.

- If a loose body is present, then there may be locking or clicking of the joint with associated instability.
- However, patients may not present until later in life with osteoarthritis.

Investigations

Initial imaging is with an x-ray, but computed tomography (CT) and magnetic resonance imaging (MRI) may be needed to fully assess the lesion.

Treatment

- If the affected segment is stable, i.e. undisplaced with intact cartilage, then treatment is conservative with a recommendation of reducing the offending sport for 6–12 months to allow time for recovery.
- If the segment is unstable with clear demarcated borders, then treatment depends on the size of the lesion.
  - If small, then removal via arthroscopy is indicated, however larger lesions may be amenable to being screwed or pinned back into place.

9.4 PATELLO-FEMORAL DISORDERS

RECURRENT DISLOCATION OF THE PATELLA

Epidemiology
The patient is often, but not always a female teenager.

Aetiology
- Due to the slight valgus angulation of the normal knee, there is a tendency for the patella to be pulled laterally during quadriceps contraction.
- This lateral movement is restricted by a number of mechanisms:
  - The patella tracks along the trochlear groove during extension.
  - The trochlear groove has a high lateral wall.
  - Several strong stabilizing medial structures, including vastus medialis prevent excessive lateral displacement.
- Dislocation of the patella may therefore occur when the knee is in slight flexion so that the extensor muscles are relaxed and a sharp twisting movement occurs.
- It is an injury seen in both dancers and those playing field sports, such as rugby, though if underlying pathology is severe enough dislocation or subluxation may occur during normal day-to-day activity.
- In most cases, there is an underlying reason for the dislocation. These include:
  - A shallow trochlear groove
  - High riding patella (patella alta)
  - A small patella
  - Ligamentous laxity
  - Valgus deformity of the knee.

Clinical features
- In first time dislocations, the patient is likely to complain of a tearing sensation and severe pain in the knee.
- They may describe feeling that their knee went out of place.
- The knee joint will immediately swell and is likely to be particularly tender over the medial side and the patient is unable to walk comfortably.
- Most patella dislocations will spontaneously return to the correct position, but if not they can often be eased back in to place while gently extending the knee.
- Between 15 and 20% of patients suffering a patella dislocation will redislocate.

Lower limb

Investigations

Anteroposterior (AP), lateral and skyline view x-rays: 5% of dislocations will also have an associated osteochondral fracture.

Treatment

- Initial treatment is to ensure that the patella is reduced.
- Following a short period of immobilization, intensive physiotherapy is required to build up the strength of the vastus medialus oblique muscle to reduce the risk of further dislocation.
- If recurrent dislocation becomes a problem, then surgical intervention should be considered.

MICRO-print

Following a dislocation of the patella, clinical signs are subtle but are likely to include:

- A positive apprehension test. This is where moving the patient's patella laterally while their knee is relaxed in slight flexion causes an uncomfortable sensation that dislocation is going to reoccur.
- Wasting of the quadriceps muscles. After any swelling of the knee, these muscles rapidly waste and therefore intensive physiotherapy to restore their bulk is very important.

OSGOOD SCHLATTER'S DISEASE

Epidemiology

Osgood Schlatter's disease is common in adolescence and more common in males. It may be bilateral and affects those engaged in strenuous exercise.

Aetiology

The underlying mechanism is from recurrent traction of the apophysis around the site of patella insertion.

Clinical features

Patients will complain of pain and a lump after exercise that is situated over the tibial tuberosity. The pain is often worse when going upstairs.

Investigations

Radiographs will show the prominence over the tibial tuberosity, however, the diagnosis is a clinical one.

Treatment

Treatment is with rest and restriction of the offending activity for several months.

The prominences over the tibial tuberosity will remain but do not cause any further trouble.

SEPTIC ARTHRITIS

Definition
Septic arthritis is defined as bacterial infection within the joint space.

Aetiology and pathophysiology
The causative organism is usually *Staphylococcus aureus*.

Clinical features
Septic arthritis presents as a warm, painful, swollen knee.

Investigations
White cell count (WCC) and C-reactive protein (CRP) are elevated. Aspiration of the joint may reveal pus in the joint space. This should be sent for microscopy, culture and sensitivity.

Management
Systemic antibiotics should be started urgently and the joint washed out in theatre.

MICRO-print
If a prosthetic joint is present, always contact an orthopaedic surgeon as joint aspiration should always be performed in theatre and not on the ward due to the high risk of an infected prosthesis.

9.5 SWELLINGS AROUND THE KNEE

POPLITEAL CYST

Epidemiology
Popliteal cyst is usually seen in elderly patients with osteoarthritis or rheumatoid arthritis.

Aetiology
The popliteal cyst is caused by bulging of the posterior capsule and synovial herniation. They are also known as Baker's cysts (after Dr William Baker who first described them).

Lower limb

Clinical features

- Lump found posteriorly in the midline usually at the level of the joint.
- Fluctuant swelling.
- May be tense on extension and soft on flexion (Foucher's sign).

Investigations

- In the first instance ultrasound scan (USS). This is also useful for excluding the presence of a deep vein thrombosis (DVT).
- MRI may be needed if more detailed views are required or there is diagnostic uncertainty.

Treatment

- A conservative approach may result in spontaneous resolution.
- Arthroscopic surgery may be useful in treating an underlying knee arthropathy, which can lead to resolution.
- If conservative or arthroscopic methods fail, then open surgery may be necessary.

SEMIMEMBRANOSUS BURSA

A posterior swelling, this involves enlargement of the normal bursa found between the semimembranosus and medial head of the gastrocnemius.
It is usually fluctuant and communicates with the knee joint.

POPLITEAL ANEURYSM

Epidemiology

Popliteal aneurysms affect the elderly.

Aetiology

It is the most common limb aneurysm and may be bilateral.

Clinical features

- May be painful
- Pulsatile
- Palpable mass.

Investigations

USS of both legs.

Treatment

Treatment is by careful monitoring or surgical repair.

MICRO-facts

Although most posterior lumps can be left alone, you may wish to aspirate some to confirm a diagnosis. However, it is vital that any posterior lump is carefully felt and that if unsure an ultrasound scan or MRI is sought beforehand to ensure you are not about to stick a needle into an aneurysm.

PREPATELLAR BURSITIS

- Also known as 'housemaid's knee'.
- Fluctuant swelling located on the front of the knee over the patella.
- Develops as a result of recurrent friction between the patella and the skin.
- Most commonly found in those working on their knees without protection, e.g. carpenters.
- Treatment for prepatellar bursitis is with firm bandaging and avoiding kneeling without protective pads. The bursa may require aspiration.

INFRAPATELLAR BURSITIS

- Also known as 'clergyman's knee'.
- This occurs below the patella and over the patellar tendon, i.e. just distal to prepatellar bursitis.
- Occurs in individuals who work on their knees.
- Treatment for infrapatellar bursitis is with firm bandaging and avoiding kneeling without protective pads. The bursa may require aspiration.

9.6 TRAUMA

KNEE DISLOCATION

Epidemiology
- Uncommon
- Can affect any age.

Aetiology
Knee dislocation involves large enough forces to tear at least two of the major ligaments in the knee.

Clinical features
- There is gross deformity, as well as severe bruising and swelling.
- The main complication with dislocation of the knee is of neurovascular injury.

Lower limb

- The popliteal artery is at risk of being torn and therefore careful monitoring of vascular status is needed.
- The lateral popliteal nerve may be injured and therefore distal sensation and movement should be tested.

Investigations
- CT scan
- Ankle brachial pressure index (ABPI) and angiography if any abnormality.

Treatment
- Urgent reduction of the joint under anaesthetic is required to reduce the risk of further injury, but vascular surgical help should be immediately available.
- If there is any delay in diagnosing a neurovascular injury of this type, then there is a very real risk that the patient will require amputation.
- Surgical reconstruction.

ANTERIOR CRUCIATE LIGAMENT INJURY

The ACL consists of two fibre bundles which run from the intercondylar region of the distal femur to the proximal tibia. The ACL prevents the tibia from moving forward in relation to the femur.

Epidemiology
- Affects the active population, most commonly aged 15–45 years.
- Seventy per cent are involved in a sporting activity.

Aetiology
- Injury to the ACL is very common during sporting activities.
- Direct trauma is not necessarily required and may occur as the patient lands from a jump or pushes off when side-stepping.
- It may also occur following a twisting or impact injury from behind while the foot is planted on the ground.

Clinical features
- The patient will report hearing a snap or pop as the ligament fails and the patient may have fallen to the ground unable to carry on with the activity.
- There is often immediate swelling of the knee (there is a blood vessel within the ACL).

Investigations
- Careful clinical examination will reveal the injury.
- Plain radiograph, MRI and CT will rule out any associated injuries and enable planning for surgery.

Treatment

- Either conservative with drainage of the haemarthrosis.
- This is then followed by physiotherapy.
- The other option is for surgical reconstruction using either autologous tendon transfer such as from the hamstring or patella tendon, or tendon taken from a cadaver.
- Surgery is also followed by intensive physiotherapy.

POSTERIOR CRUCIATE LIGAMENT INJURY

Mechanism of injury/aetiology

- The PCL originates deep in the distal femur and attaches to the posterior surface of the tibia.
- The PCL restricts posterior movement of the tibia relative to the femur.
- This injury occurs in a flexed knee, when the tibia is forced backwards, such as in a head-on collision in a car or a tackle from the front to the knee in American football.

Clinical features

- Pain
- Rapid swelling
- Feeling of instability within the knee joint.

Treatment

- If it is an isolated PCL injury, then most patients do very well with conservative management with a period in a knee splint.
- Arthroscopic repair is available if surgical intervention is needed.

Complications

- Long-term knee pain
- Instability
- Osteoarthritis.

MEDIAL COLLATERAL AND LATERAL COLLATERAL LIGAMENT INJURY

- Complete tears of the medial collateral ligament (MCL) are often seen in conjunction with ACL injuries.
- MCL injury occurs after a valgus force, but most do not require surgery.
- Lateral collateral ligament (LCL) tears occur following a blow to the medial side of the knee, putting a varus force through the joint.
- Isolated injuries of the LCL are uncommon and if seen you should always look for cruciate ligament damage and test for common peroneal nerve damage which may have been stretched or torn during the injury.

Lower limb

MENISCAL INJURY

Mechanism of injury/aetiology

- Damage to either or both medial and lateral menisci is associated with ligamentous injury, although relatively minor twisting incidents may result in a meniscal tear.
- Damage to the medial meniscus is more common.
- Types of meniscal tear include (Fig. 9.4):
  - Longitudinal tear
  - Parrot beak tear (rupture of the central edge)
  - Bucket handle tear.

Clinical features

- Unlike ligament damage, swelling occurs slowly after the injury occurs.
- Typically, the patient will describe a pattern of recurrent locking with periods of normality.
- This locking is caused by the mobile fragment catching in the joint (thereby preventing movement).

Diagnosis and treatment

- Plain x-ray followed by MRI allows diagnosis in most cases.
- If symptoms are problematic, arthroscopy can be carried out with the torn portion being removed at the same time (meniscectomy).

Complications

- The menisci form an important part of the load-bearing mechanism in the knee.
- Damage to the menisci may result in increased pressure being transmitted through the bony articular surfaces dramatically increasing the risk of early onset osteoarthritis.
- If osteoarthritis is already present, then it will rapidly progress.

MICRO-print

O'Donoghue's triad is the combination of damage to the following structures occurs:

- Anterior cruciate ligament
- Medial collateral ligament
- Medial meniscus

This occurs when a valgus force is applied to the knee when the foot is fixed to the ground and is twisted into external rotation.

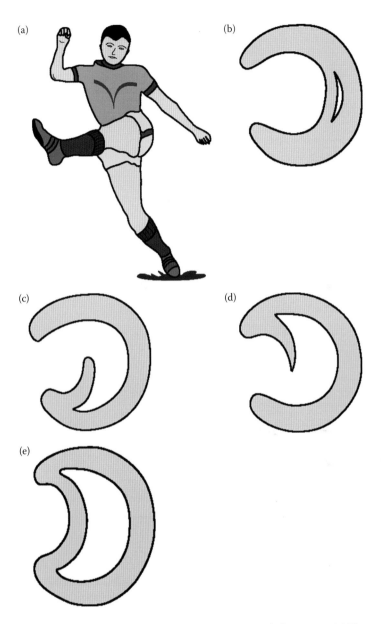

Fig. 9.4 Types of medial meniscal tear (a–e). **Torn medial meniscus (a)** The meniscus is usually torn by a twisting force with the knee bent and taking weight; the initial split **(b)** may extend anteriorly **(c)**, posteriorly **(d)** or both ways to create a 'bucket-handle' tear **(e)**. Reproduced with permission from Solomon L, Warwick D, Nayagam S (eds.). *Apley's System of Orthopaedics and Fractures*, 9th edn. London: Hodder Arnold, 2010.

PATELLA FRACTURES AND DAMAGE TO THE EXTENSOR MECHANISM

Mechanism of injury/aetiology

- Fractures to the patella can occur as a result of direct violence, such as in a car crash or falling on to the edge of a hard surface.
- Fractures to the patella and extensor mechanism may also occur by indirect forces, such as in sudden muscular contraction, causing avulsion fractures.

Clinical features

- The patient will most likely be unable to extend the knee or straight leg raise.
- There may be a palpable gap above or below the patella.

Treatment

- If there is a comminuted fracture of the patella (stellate fracture), then some surgeons believe a patellectomy should be considered due to the inevitable damage to the patella-femoral joint caused by the irregular patella undersurface.
- Transverse patella fractures can be fixed using K-wires to hold the two parts in place.

Complications

After any fracture to the patella, patella-femoral osteoarthritis is possible.

TIBIAL PLATEAU FRACTURES

Mechanism of injury/aetiology

- These fractures occur as a result of a varus or valgus strain on the knee combined with axial loading as seen in a fall from height.
- It is also seen when pedestrians are hit by a vehicle from the side and the femoral condyle of one side is forced on to the ipsilateral tibial condyle.
- If the forces involved are great enough, there may also be a contralateral ligament rupture or damage.

Clinical features

- Clinical presentation is of a swollen painful knee with either a varus or valgus deformity.
- X-ray may not show the true extent of the fracture and so CT is often used in these cases.

Treatment

- Treatment depends on the extent of the fracture and degree of displacement.
- Undisplaced and minimally displaced fractures of the lateral condyle may be treated conservatively with a hinge brace.

- Comminuted and markedly displaced fractures may need open reduction and internal fixation.
- Some patients with tibial plateau fractures may actually have a better outcome if they have a total knee replacement, although the results are not generally as good as in osteoarthritis.

Complications

- The major vascular complication is of damage to the popliteal artery which can lead to limb ischaemia and significant blood loss.
- There is a risk of compartment syndrome with tibial plateau fractures. If this develops or appears imminent, then the patient will need fasciotomies of the calf to relieve the pressure.
- When significant forces are involved in medial plateau fractures, there is risk of damage to the peroneal nerve and so an ankle-foot orthosis should be worn to prevent an Achilles contracture.
- There is also a risk of concomitant ligament and meniscal damage.

MICRO-facts

As with any extensive or complicated fracture, following tibial plateau fractures you must be on the look-out for any signs or symptoms of compartment syndrome.

---

10 Ankle and foot

10.1 ANKLE AND FOOT OVERVIEW

The ankle joint is a synovial hinge joint that joins the distal tibia and fibula to the talus.

This chapter simplifies the regional anatomy and reviews the common pathologies that can affect the ankle and foot. The anatomy of the ankle and foot is shown in Fig. 10.1.

> ### MICRO-facts
> **Mobility**
> The foot is arched and segmented to provide a 'shock absorbing' effect. Flexibility during movement is because of the thin fibrous capsules of the individual joints of the foot.

> ### MICRO-facts
> **Stability**
> The ankle and foot support body weight. The distal tibia and fibula are stabilized by the tibiofibular syndesmosis. The bones of the foot are shaped into arches. The ankle is supported by strong ankle ligaments (one medial and three lateral) that comprise:
> - Deltoid ligament: medial malleolus to calcaneum, talus and naviclar bones
> - Anterior talofibular ligament: lateral malleollus to talus
> - Posterior talofibular ligament: malleolar fossa to the lateral tubercle of the talus
> - Calcaneofibular ligament: lateral malleolus to lateral calcaneum.

TAKING AN 'ANKLE AND FOOT HISTORY'

- Take a systematic approach (Fig. 10.2)
- The presenting complaint: pain and/or instability
- History of presenting complaint:

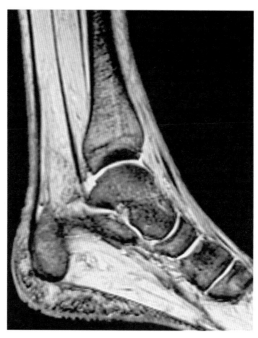

Fig. 10.1 Anatomy of the ankle and foot. Reproduced with permission from Ellis H, Logan B, Dixon A. *Human Sectional Anatomy*, 3rd edn. London: Hodder Arnold: 2007.

- SOCRATES (site, onset, character, radiation, associated findings, timing, exacerbating/relieving factors, severity)
- Impact of problem (social, domestic, work).
- Past medical history
- Family history, including congenital problems
- Drug history
- Social history
- Systems enquiry.
- The examination starts with the patient walking into the room.
  - Explain to the patient what you are about to do.
  - Both of the patient's legs must be exposed from the knees to toes.
  - Do not cause undue pain or discomfort.
  - Compare sides.
  - Examine the hip and knee joints.
  - A complete neurovascular assessment is essential.
  - Do not forget to look at the patient's shoes.

ANKLE AND FOOT EXAMINATION

- With the patient standing:

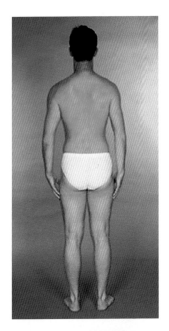
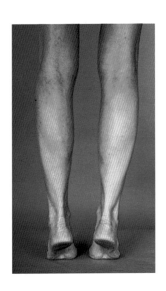
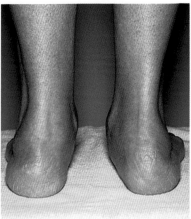
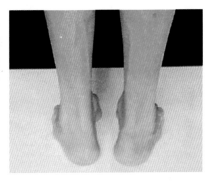

Fig. 10.2 Examination of feet with patient standing. Look at the patient as a whole, first from in front and from behind. (a, b) The heels are normally in slight valgus and should invert equally when a patient stands on his/her toes. (c) This patient has flat feet (pes planus), while the patient in (d) has the opposite deformity, varus heels and an abnormally high longitudinal arch – pes cavus (e). From the front you can again notice (f) the dropped longitudinal arch in the patient with pes planus, as well as the typical deformities of bilateral hallux valgus and overriding toes. (g) Corns on the top of the toes are common. Reproduced with permission from Solomon L, Warwick D, Nayagam S (eds.). *Apley's System of Orthopaedics and Fractures*, 9th edn. London: Hodder Arnold, 2010.

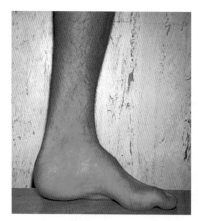
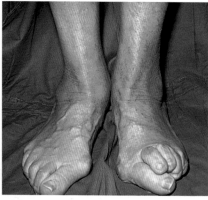

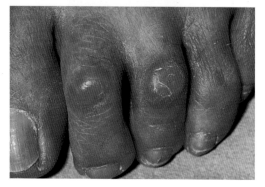

Fig. 10.2 (*Continued*)

- With both legs exposed inspect the front, side and back of the patient. The heels are normally in equal plantar grade and in slight valgus position.
- Ask the patient to walk a few metres, turn and walk back towards you.
- With the patient supine or sitting with their foot on the examiner's lap, inspect for deformities, swellings and foot callosities.
- Palpation
  - Do not forget skin temperature! Use the back of your hand. This is a useful indication of joint inflammation.
  - Feel for any lumps and deformities that might not be apparent on inspection.

MICRO-facts

There are specific terms for the position of the feet/toes:
- Plantigrade: normal position: the sole is at right angles to the leg
- Calcaneus: dorsiflexed (foot up)

continued...

continued...

- Equinus: plantar flexed (foot down)
- Cavus: high arch
- Planus: flat foot
- Hallux valgus: big toe deviated laterally.
- 'Hammer'/'claw' toes: interphalangeal joint(s) flexed.

- Movement
  - Use a systematic approach to assess each joint of the ankle and foot. Look for an active range of movement. Elicit the full range for the patient.
  - Repeat movements passively; feel for crepitus. Explain the proposed movements before you start the examination and try not to cause discomfort:
    - Ankle joint: test plantar/dorsiflexion
    - Subtalar joint: test inversion and eversion
    - Mid-tarsal joints: move the tarsus in dorsi and plantar flexion while holding the hind foot static
    - Toes: test movements at the inter-phalangeal and metatarso-phalangeal joints
    - Remember to palpate the sole for local tenderness.

MICRO-facts

Always complete the examination with a neurovascular evaluation:
- Sensation and power can be tested at the same time as palpation and movement.
- Posterior tibial pulse; push inwards and feel against the posterior aspect of the medial malleollus.
- Dorsalis pedis pulse: with your fingers parallel and immediately lateral to the tendon of extensor hallucis longus.

IMAGING

There are several routine radiographs that must be requested depending upon the ankle/foot pathology being sought:
- Anteroposterior
- Lateral
- Standing
- With joint stressed
- Computed tomography (CT) scan is used for complex fractures
- Ultrasound and magnetic resonance imaging (MRI) are used for soft tissue abnormalities.

Lower limb

Table 10.1 **Possible ankle and foot pathology.**

SITE	POSSIBLE ANKLE AND FOOT PATHOLOGY
Heel	Plantar fasciitis, Achilles tendon rupture
Midfoot	Flat foot, pes cavus
Forefoot	Callosities, diabetes mellitus (DM), rheumatoid arthritis (RA)
Big toe	Hallux valgus, hallux rigidus, callosities, gout, DM, RA
Other toes	Hammer toe, claw toes, DM, RA

SITE VERSUS ANKLE AND FOOT PATHOLOGY

Your main clue in diagnosing ankle and foot pathology will be the site of the patient's pain (**Table 10.1**). Pain at various sites and the related most common pathology is set out in the table (note that trauma and secondary osteoarthritis (OA) are common causes at all sites).

10.2 CLUB FOOT

DEFINITION

Club foot is defined as a plantar grade inverted foot (Fig. 10.3).

AETIOLOGY

Club foot is a common congenital condition and is multifactorial in aetiology.

CLINICAL FEATURES

- Foot points down and inwards (equinovarus).
- In 30%, the condition is bilateral.
- Note. Club foot can be associated with spina bifida and congenital. Dislocation of the hip. These conditions must be excluded.
- Further investigations depend upon the clinical findings.

MANAGEMENT

- Most cases are treated by manipulation and plaster of Paris stabilization until the foot is corrected to neutral alignment (Ponseti method).
- Severe cases may require surgical intervention, i.e. tendon release, transposition and/or lengthening.
- Relapse or late club foot may require external fixation (with an Ilizarov frame).

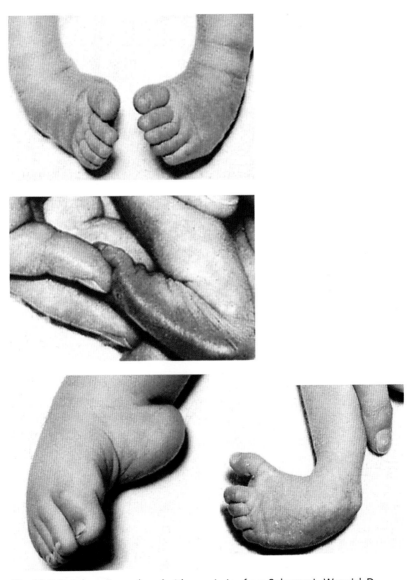

Fig. 10.3 Club foot. Reproduced with permission from Solomon L, Warwick D, Nayagam S (eds.). *Apley's System of Orthopaedics and Fractures*, 9th edn. London: Hodder Arnold, 2010.

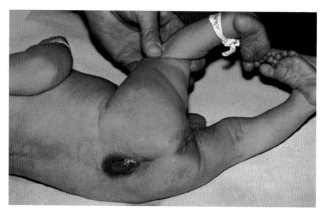

Fig. 10.3 (*Continued*)

10.3 PES PLANUS (FLAT FEET)

DEFINITION

The medial aspect of the foot is in contact with the ground when weight bearing.

EPIDEMIOLOGY

Flat feet mainly affects younger children and teenagers.

CLINICAL FEATURES

There are two types: flexible and rigid:
- Flexible flat feet: usually asymptomatic
- Rigid flat feet: often painful as caused by coalition of bone between the calcaneum, talus and navicular.

Clinical tip: Ask the patient to stand on tiptoes. Flexible flat feet will show heel inversion without lower anterior compartment spasm.

MANAGEMENT

Treatment should exclude inflammatory conditions:
- Flexible asymptomatic flat feet are usually self-correcting. Provide reassurance.
- Rigid flat feet may require splinting and/or removal of coalition bone.

10.4 PES CAVUS (HIGH ARCHED FEET)

DEFINITION

Pes cavus is defined as high arched feet associated with 'claw' toes.

CLINICAL FEATURES

- Metatarsals are pushed downwards into the sole.
- Callosities may be present.

MANAGEMENT

Custom-made shoes normally suffice. If there is fixed deformity and pain, surgical tissue releases ± arthrodesis.

10.5 HALLUX VALGUS

DEFINITION

Hallus valgus is defined by lateral deviation of the hallux with 'bunion' deformity. It is the most common musculoskeletal deformity.

EPIDEMIOLOGY

It mainly affects older females.

MANAGEMENT

Treatment is by bunion excision or osteotomy to correct position.

10.6 HALLUX RIGIDUS

DEFINITION

Hallux rigidus is defined by first metatarsophalangeal joint stiffness with pain. It is associated with most commonly with OA also chronic gout, pseudogout and post-trauma.

CLINICAL FEATURES

The clinical picture is of pain and reduced dorsiflexion.

MANAGEMENT

Treatment is with rocker-sole shoes, arthrodesis (fusion) or removal of osteophytes.

10.7 HAMMER AND CLAW TOES

DEFINITION

Hammer and claw toes are defined as fixed flexion deformity of one ('hammer') or all toes ('claw').

CLINICAL FEATURES

The clinical features are painful corns on the dorsal aspect of the affected toe due to pressure.

MANAGEMENT

Treatment is with metatarsal supports and joint fusion.

10.8 PLANTAR FASCIITIS

DEFINITION

Plantar fasciitis is defined as local pain under the plantar aspect of the central heel.

INVESTIGATION

Lateral x-ray may show a bony (calcaneal) spur. This is not proven to be the cause of the foot pain.

MANAGEMENT

Treatment involves rest, heel pads, non-steroidal anti-inflammatory drugs (NSAIDs) or local injection of corticosteroid.

10.9 ACHILLES TENDON RUPTURE

MECHANISM OF INJURY

The tendon ruptures when the foot pushes forcefully against the ground, e.g. running uphill.

ASSESSMENT

Acute pain described: 'feels like I've been kicked in the calf'; located 5 cm superior to the tendon insertion.

Clinical test: Simmond's test

With patient prone, squeeze their calf:
- Tendon ruptured: foot does not move.
- Tendon intact: foot plantar flexes.

MANAGEMENT

- Non-surgical: plaster cast for 6–8 weeks
- Surgical: suture repair either open or percutaneously.

10.10 FRACTURES AND DISLOCATIONS

MECHANISM OF INJURY

Commonly, there is a history of ankle twisting and acute severe pain, and the patient is unable to weight bear.

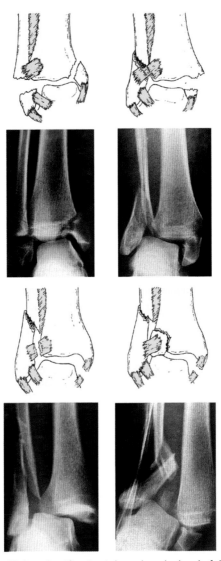

Fig. 10.4 The Danis-Weber classification is based on the level of the fibular fracture. Type A – a fibular fracture below the syndesmosis and an oblique fracture of the medial malleolus (caused by forced supination and adduction of the foot). **(b)** Type B – fracture at the syndesmosis, often associated with disruption of the anterior fibres of the tibiofibular ligament and fracture of the posterior and/or medial malleolus, or disruption of the medial ligament (caused by forced supination and external rotation). **(c)** Type C – a fibular fracture above the syndesmosis; the tibiofibular ligament must be torn, or else **(d)** the ligament avulses a small piece of the tibia. Here, again, there must also be disruption on the medial side of the joint – either a medial malleolar fracture or rupture of the deltoid ligament. Reproduced with permission from Solomon L, Warwick D, Nayagam S (eds.). *Apley's System of Orthopaedics and Fractures*, 9th edn. London: Hodder Arnold, 2010.

ASSESSMENT

Assessment follows classifications using: Danis-Weber, Salter-Harris and Lis-Franc. A clinical diagnosis of an ankle fracture can be made using the Ottawa ankle rules.

- Danis-Weber: three types (Fig. 10.4):
  - Malleollar fracture distal to syndesmosis
  - Malleolar fracture at the syndesmosis
  - Malleolar fracture proximal to the syndesmosis.

As shown on the figure, A is more stable than B and C and is usually managed with plaster cast. B and C require internal fixation

- Salter-Harris: fractures of the tibia and fibula in children. There are nine types. I to V are the most common:
  - Type I. An epiphyseal slip
  - Type II. Fracture through physis and metaphysis
  - Type III. Fracture through physis and epiphysis
  - Type IV. Fracture through physis, metaphysis and epiphysis
  - Type V. Compression fracture of the physis.

- Lisfranc:
  - Tarso-metatarsal fracture dislocation.
  - Important to exclude (often missed) in polytrauma patients as can cause compartment syndrome of the medial foot.
  - X-ray: Widened space between second metatarsal base and medial cuneiform bone.
  - Patient will often have bruising on the plantar surface of the foot.
  - Treatment is by prompt and accurate reduction ± ORIF (open reduction, internal fixation).

MICRO-print
The Ottawa Ankle and Foot Rules
Useful in clinical emergencies when examining the ankle as the rules reduce the need for unnecessary x-rays. When palpating the patient's foot, one of the following is an indication for suspecting a fracture and that an x-ray is required:
- Local medial malleolar tenderness
- Local lateral malleolar tenderness
- Patient unable to weight bear or take four steps
- Fifth metatarsal styloid tenderness
- Navicular tenderness.

For information on osteoarthritis and gout, see Chapter 16, Non-inflammatory arthroses and Chapter 15, Crystal arthropathies, respectively. Classically, rheumatoid arthritis (RA) is a small joint polyarthropathy and affects the feet almost as often as the hands (see Chapter 11, Rheumatoid arthritis, for more information).

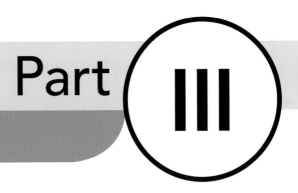

Part III

Rheumatology

11 Rheumatoid arthritis

11.1 RHEUMATOID ARTHRITIS

DEFINITION

Rheumatoid arthritis (RA) is a chronic, multi-system, inflammatory disease. The characteristic feature is polyarthritis, mainly affecting the small joints of the hands and feet, although extra-articular features may be present.

EPIDEMIOLOGY

- Females > male (3:1).
- The disease can start at any age, but is usually between the ages of 40 and 60 years.
- Men tend to get the disease after 45 years old but for women, the incidence rises until 45 years old and then remains the same.
- The economic cost of the disease in the UK reaches into the billions every year.
- In men and women, life expectancy is shortened by seven and three years, respectively. Several factors contribute to this, in particular an increased risk of cardiovascular disease.

AETIOLOGY

The exact aetiology of RA is unknown, but several theories have been postulated:
- **Genetics**. The presence of human leukocyte antigen (HLA) genes appears to be involved. HLA-DR4 increases the risk of developing the disease and affects the severity.
- **Environment**. It is thought that certain lifestyle habits may be involved, but no causative factors have been found.

PATHOGENESIS

The root cause of RA is poorly understood, despite much research in the area. Activated macrophages within synovium produce T-lymphocytes which activate other macrophages, producing cytokines including:
- Tumour necrosis factor-alpha (TNF-α)
- Interleukin-1 (IL-1).

These cytokines then initiate an inflammatory response which leads to:
- Bone and cartilage destruction
- Synovitis
- The production of antibodies including:
  - Rheumatoid factor (RF)
  - Antibodies to cyclic citrullinated peptides (anti-CCP), which are found in the serum of the majority of patients with RA.

MICRO-facts

Anti-CCP is both more sensitive and specific than RF throughout the course of RA.

CLINICAL FEATURES

Articular

- Typically, symmetrical, polyarthritic small joint disease is present.
- Pain, stiffness (worse in the morning) and swelling of the involved joints.
- Onset is typically insidious over weeks or months and the patient may be able to identify one joint that initially became affected, preceding multi-joint involvement.
- Patients may also present with only one or two joints involved: in this case the knee or shoulder are common sites.
- The classical picture is of red, warm, tender and swollen small joints of the hands and feet, but not in the distal interphalangeal joints, as these are not synovial joints.
- Patients may complain of difficulty with activities of daily living, such as doing up buttons.
- Only synovial joints are affected (this may include the atlanto-axial joints in the cervical spine, leading to instability).
- Stiffness tends to ease the more the joint is used.

The classification criteria for rheumatoid arthritis can be found in Fig. 11.1, while Fig. 11.2 shows the four stages of joint pathology.

MICRO-facts

RA hand signs are a common examination question (Fig. 11.3):
- Ulnar deviation of the fingers distal to the MCP joint
- Boutonnière deformity of the fingers (Fig. 11.4b)
- Swan neck deformity (Fig. 11.4a)
- Radial deviation of the wrist
- Z-shaped thumb
- Knuckle subluxation (dropped finger)
- Wrist subluxation
- Elbow nodules

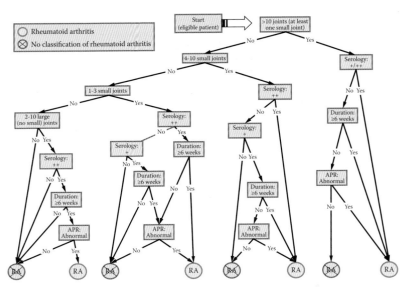

Fig. 11.1 Rheumatoid arthritis classification criteria. Reproduced with permission from Aletaha D, Neogi T, Silman AJ et al. Rheumatoid arthritis classification criteria: an American College of Rheumatology/European League Against Rheumatism collaborative initiative. *Annals of the Rheumatic Diseases* 2010; **69**: 1580.

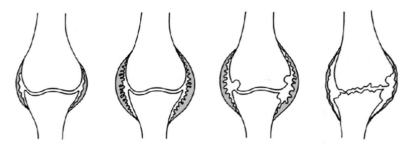

Fig. 11.2 Four stages of pathological changes found in rheumatoid arthritis. (a) The normal joint. (b) Stage 1. Synovitis and joint swelling. (c) Stage 2. Early joint destruction with periarticular erosions. (d) Stage 3 advanced joint destruction and deformity. Reproduced with permission from Solomon L, Warwick D, Nayagam S. *Apley's System of Orthopaedics and Fractures*, 8th edn. London: Hodder Arnold, 2001.

Extra-articular

- Systemic symptoms: fever, fatigue, malaise, weight loss
- Musculoskeletal:
    - osteoporotic fractures
    - tenosynovitis and bursitis
    - rupture of tendons and ligaments
- Pulmonary:
    - pleuritis with pleural effusion (exudative)

Rheumatology

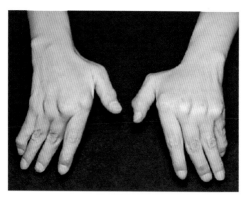

Fig. 11.3 A hand showing the classical signs of rheumatoid arthritis. Reproduced with permission from Solomon L, Warwick D, Nayagam S. *Apley's System of Orthopaedics and Fractures*, 8th edn. London: Hodder Arnold, 2001.

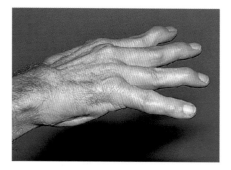 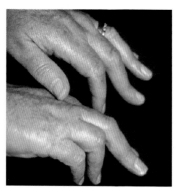

Fig. 11.4 Swan-neck deformity (a) and boutonnière deformity (b) of the fingers. Reproduced with permission from Solomon L, Warwick D, Nayagam S. *Apley's System of Orthopaedics and Fractures*, 8th edn. London: Hodder Arnold, 2001.

- nodules
- fibrosis
- Cardiovascular:
  - pericarditis ± pericardial effusion
  - ↑ cardiovascular mortality
  - Myocarditis
  - Vasculitis
- Ocular:
  - keratoconjunctivitis sicca
  - scleritis
  - episcleritis

- Neurological:
  - mononeuritis multiplex
  - cervical subluxation causing pain and neurological symptoms
  - nerve entrapment, e.g. carpal tunnel syndrome
- Infections:
  - septic arthritis may occur, especially in prosthetic joints
  - immunosuppressive drugs used in RA predispose to infection
- Skin:
  - palmar erythema
  - nodules
  - Raynaud's phenomenon
- Amyloidosis:
  - involving skin, kidneys, heart, liver and the gastrointestinal tract
- Felty's syndrome:
  - RA with splenomegaly and leukopenia
  - These manifestations increase the risk of infections and lymphadenopathy
  - Anaemia and thrombocytopaenia may result from splenomegaly.

MICRO-facts

Another examiner's favourite: why do patients with RA get anaemia?
There are several reasons:

- Anaemia of chronic disease
- Felty's syndrome
- Autoimmune haemolysis
- Drug induced
  - Iron-deficiency anaemia due to non-steroidal anti-inflammatory drugs (NSAIDs)-induced gastritis
  - Bone marrow suppression due to disease-modifying antirheumatic drugs (DMARDs).

INVESTIGATIONS

Blood tests

Full blood count (FBC), C-reactive protein (CRP), erythrocyte sedimentation rate (ESR), plasma viscosity, rheumatoid factor, anti-cyclic citrullinated peptide (anti-CCP) antibodies.

MICRO-reference

National Rheumatoid Arthritis Society. Disease activity score. Accessed August 2012. Available from: www.nras.org.uk/about_rheumatoid_arthritis/established_disease/disease_activity_score_das/default.aspx

Radiographic imaging

- X-rays of affected joints
- Ultrasound or magnetic resonance image (MRI) for more specific imaging of joints
- High resolution computed tomography of the chest for patients with pulmonary symptoms.

Aspiration of synovial fluid

- Valuable if diagnosis uncertain due to an atypical presentation or joint infection is suspected.

MICRO-print

People without RA may have rheumatoid factor in their serum, especially people who have other conditions such as tuberculosis (TB), sarcoidosis and leprosy.

RESULTS

Table 11.1 shows expected results following investigation of patients with suspected rheumatoid arthritis.

MICRO-case

Mrs. Articular is a 42-year-old woman who has just been diagnosed with rheumatoid arthritis that is present bilaterally and symmetrically in her hands and wrists. There is evidence to suggest that she has an aggressive form of the disease as she had a high titre of rheumatoid factor in her serum. Today, the rheumatologist wants to take some x-rays of her hands to see if there are any changes present due to the disease. Changes are seen on the radiographs.

Points to consider
Rheumatoid arthritis can cause: decreased joint space, peri-articular erosions, juxta-articular osteopenia, juxta-articular osteoporosis and tissue swelling.

DIFFERENTIAL DIAGNOSES

- Viral arthritis: hepatitis B and C
- Septic arthritis
- Gout/pseudogout
- Psoriatic arthritis
- Connective tissue disease, systemic lupus erythematosus (SLE), Sjögren's syndrome
- Leukaemia
- Lymphoma

Table 11.1 Results of investigations in patients with rheumatoid arthritis (RA).

INVESTIGATION	RESULT IN PATIENTS WITH RA
Full blood count (FBC)	
Haemoglobin	↓
Platelets	↑
Leukocytes	↓
Erythrocyte sedimentation rate (ESR)	↑
C-reactive protein (CRP)	↑
Plasma viscosity	↑
Rheumatoid factor	Present (70–80% of RA patients) versus not present (20–30% of RA patients)
Anti-CCP	Usually present
X-rays	Decreased joint space
	Peri-articular erosions
	Juxta-articular osteopenia/porosis
	Tissue swelling
Synovial fluid	↑ protein
	↑ leukocytes
	No organisms
	No crystals

MANAGEMENT

- Good management involves a range of modalities tailored to the individual patient.
- Early intervention improves prognosis.

Information

- It is important that patients can get the information they want on their disease.
- Patients need to be taught about their disease and have access to good information.
- Arthritis Research UK produces many information leaflets available in clinics and online.

Rheumatology

Physiotherapy

- Physiotherapists can advise patients on exercises they can do to keep their mobility and independence at a maximum.

Happy feet

- Podiatrists and chiropodists can make sure patients are wearing appropriate shoes, give orthoses and manage problems with the feet.

Occupational therapy

- Occupational therapists can show patients how to carry out activities of daily living in an appropriate fashion for the patient.
- They can also splint joints and give aids and adaptations for the patient's home.

Surgical options

- Orthopaedic surgeons can perform a range of surgical therapies for patients with severe RA.

Regular appointments

- The rheumatologist will usually be in charge of monitoring the patient and ensuring they are following the appropriate treatment.

Medications

- Simple analgesia, such as paracetamol, can be prescribed to alleviate pain.
- NSAIDs provide pain relief and decrease inflammation.
- Steroids are usually given as intra-articular injections, short oral courses or as intramuscular boluses for very active disease. They are effective in reducing pain and inflammation.
- DMARDs:
  - Do as their name suggests; reduce joint damage by slowing the disease.
  - The downside to these drugs is that they can take up to six months to have an effect.
  - They can also produce some severe side effects, such as bone marrow suppression, renal impairment, oral ulcers, rash, gastro-intestinal (GI) upset, proteinuria and deranged liver enzymes.
  - Examples of common DMARDs include methotrexate, sulfasalazine, hydroxychloroquine, leflunomide, gold and azathioprine. Combination therapy is recommended.
- Biologic agents:
  - Anti-TNF-α:
  - Adalimumab, etanercept, infliximab, certolizumab and golimumab.

- Although very effective, these drugs are powerful immunosuppressants and extremely expensive and so there are stringent guidelines for prescribing.
- Other biologic agents:
  - An increasing range of other monoclonal antibodies are available for treatment of severe RA resistant to DMARDs and anti-TNF drugs
  - Rituximab is a monoclonal antibody against CD20 which is present on B cells.
  - Abatacept is an inhibitor of T-cell co-stimulatory molecules.
  - Tocilizumab is an inhibitor of IL-6. It is usually used when other medications have failed to have an effect.

PROGNOSIS

- RA is a chronic disease. The goal is to suppress symptoms and to achieve remission. There is no cure.
- The majority of patients with RA will have moderate disease which will exhibit periods of flare up and remission.
- Poor prognosis can be identified by factors such as erosions on x-ray, high levels of rheumatoid factor and rheumatoid nodules.
- Cardiovascular disease risk is increased and so life expectancy is reduced.

MICRO-case

Mr. Synovium is a 50-year-old businessman who presents to his GP with pain in the balls of his feet which are also red and swollen. He says that they are really painful to walk on when he wakes up in the morning, but they ease the more he moves them. After investigations, he is diagnosed with rheumatoid arthritis.

Points to consider

- Appropriate investigations for RA include: FBC, CRP, ESR, plasma viscosity, rheumatoid factor and anti-cyclic citrullinated peptide (anti-CCP) antibodies.
- It should be noted that anti-CCP antibodies have a higher degree of sensitivity and specificity than rheumatoid factor but both tests together give high diagnostic specificity.
- An x-ray of the man's feet may show peri-articular osteopenia or early erosions.

12 Connective tissue diseases

12.1 SYSTEMIC LUPUS ERYTHEMATOSUS

DEFINITION

Systemic lupus erythematosus (SLE) is a multisystem inflammatory disease with first presentation usually between the ages of 15 and 40 years.

AETIOLOGY

The aetiology is multifactoral and also can be iatrogenic, e.g. medications such as hydrazaline.

PATHOLOGY

- Dysfunction of the immune system with increased activity of B cells
- Dysfunctional cell mediated immunity
- Poor clearance of immune complexes from tissues.

CLINICAL FEATURES

- These are diverse as it is a multisystem disease.
- General clinical features are weight loss, fever and fatigue.
- Musculoskeletal features include polyarticular arthritis and myalgia.
- Other system features include:
    - Butterfly rash
    - Photosensitivity
    - Alopecia
    - Anaemia/thrombocytopenia
    - Raynaud's phenomenon
    - Myocarditis/Pericarditis
    - Aortic valve lesions
    - Glomerulonephritis (all types).

Note: This list is by no means exclusive and any organ can be affected.

INVESTIGATIONS

- Full blood count (FBC)
- Urea and electrolytes (U&Es)

- Erythrocyte sedimentation rate (ESR) (likely to be raised in an SLE flare up)
- C-reactive protein (CRP)
- Tissue biopsies
- Autoantibodies, such as anti-nuclear antibody (ANA), anti-phospholipid, anti-double stranded DNA (high specificity for SLE), anti-cardiolipin, anti-Smith (anti-Sm)
- Complement C3 and C4 (depressed in SLE).

MANAGEMENT

- Non-steroidal anti-inflammatory drugs (NSAIDs)
- Anti-malarials
- Corticosteroids
- Disease-modifying anti-rheumatic drugs (DMARDs)
- Cytotoxics
- Anti-hypertensives (to minimize renal disease progression which is the leading cause of mortality in SLE patients).

12.2 SJÖGREN'S SYNDROME

DEFINITION

- Sjögren's syndrome is a chronic autoimmune condition characterized by destruction of the exocrine glands.

AETIOLOGY/PATHOLOGY

- Exocrine glands are infiltrated by lymphocytes causing inflammation.
- Endogenous retroviruses have been implicated in causation, but the aetiology remains unknown.

CLINICAL FEATURES

- Eyes. Dry, red, painful eyes due to the affected lacrimal glands not being able to produce tears. This can lead to keratoconjunctivitis sicca.
- Mouth. Since the salivary glands are also affected by the disease, patients may experience a dry mouth (xerostomia). Dental caries and swelling of the parotid gland are also common features.
- Exocrine glands. When affected in other parts of the body, leads to symptoms specific to the area involved. For example, a lack of exocrine gland function in the vagina will lead to vaginal dryness.
- Systemic features. Vasculitis, arthritis, lung disease, kidney disease, neurological problems, Raynaud's phenomenon and fatigue.

INVESTIGATIONS

- FBC.
- Inflammatory marker level.

- Autoantibodies: anti-Ro (anti-SSA) and anti-La (anti-SSB).
- Rheumatoid factor and antinuclear antibodies.
- Schirmer's test can be done to demonstrate lacrimal gland involvement.
- Rose-Bengal dye is put in the eye and an examination with a slit lamp is carried out to diagnose keratoconjunctivitis sicca.
- Exocrine gland biopsy classically shows a lymphocytic infiltrate.

MANAGEMENT

Treat the symptoms:
- Dry eyes: artificial tears
- Dry mouth: artificial saliva, regular drinks
- Arthritides (i.e. rheumatoid arthritis (RA) and SLE): NSAIDs and hydroxychloroquine
- Steroids may be used for severe cases.

12.3 POLYMYOSITIS

DEFINITION

Polymyositis is defined as chronic inflammation of muscles known as an inflammatory myopathy.

EPIDEMIOLOGY

This is a rare condition.

AETIOLOGY

The aetiology is unknown.

PATHOPHYSIOLOGY

- Can be due secondarily to an occult malignancy, e.g. lung or ovarian.
- Most often presents in adulthood.

CLINICAL FEATURES

- Proximal muscle weakness with early onset fatigue with walking.
- Systemic features, such as weight loss and fever.
- Muscle pain.
- The condition can affect the respiratory muscles which can lead to aspiration pneumonia and ventilatory failure.
- Pulmonary fibrosis can occur in up to 30% of patients.

INVESTIGATIONS

- Anti-Jo-1 antibodies in >65% of patients.
- Elevated serum ESR, CRP and creatine kinase (CK) are also characteristic, but not specific to polymyositis.

Rheumatology

- A muscle biopsy looking for muscle fibre necrosis, regeneration and inflammatory cell infiltration.

MANAGEMENT

- Corticosteroids. A course of high-dose prednisone, tapered according to response will often bring about a dramatic improvement.
- Maintenance steroids and immunosuppressive drugs may be useful in long-term treatment.
- A specialized exercise programme led by a physiotherapist can enhance quality of life.

MICRO-print

Dermatomyositis
- Associated with polymyositis, with similar features.
- Skin involvement:
    - Classical, 'heliotrope rash': purplish rash around the eyes
    - Gottron's papules: reddish rash over knuckles
    - Rash over 'shawl' area of back and shoulders

12.4 SYSTEMIC SCLEROSIS

DEFINITION

Rare multisystem connective tissue disorder with characteristic skin thickening – scleroderma

CLINICAL FEATURES AND MANAGEMENT

- Limited cutaneous systemic sclerosis has a better prognosis:
    - Skin involvement over face and limbs distal to elbow and knee joints only
    - Calcinosis
    - Raunaud's phenomenon
    - Esophageal/gut involvement with poor motility
    - Sclerodactyly
    - Telangectasia
    - Anti-centromere antibody associated.
- Diffuse cutaneous systemic sclerosis has a worse prognosis:
    - Skin involvement not limited, occurring also over trunk and proximal limbs
    - More severe organ involvement
    - Pulmonary fibrosis ± pulmonary hypertension (more common in limited)
    - Kidney involvement progresses to 'scleroderma renal crisis'
    - Anti SCL-70 antibody associated.

> **MICRO-print**
> **Mixed connective tissue disease**
> A mixture of features from SLE, Sjögren's, polymyositis and systemic sclerosis. Anti-ribonucleopeptide (anti-RNP) associated.

12.5 FIBROMYALGIA

DEFINITION

- Fibromyalgia is a diagnosis of exclusion.
- Patients have areas of tenderness and pain without any identifiable underlying pathology.

AETIOLOGY/PATHOLOGY

- Fibromyalgia most commonly affects women and although it can occur at any age, it usually begins between the ages of 30 and 60.
- Fibromyalgia may start following physical trauma, stress or major depression. However, there may also be no obvious trigger for the patient's symptoms.
- As no underlying pathology is found, diagnosis can be difficult. It is important therefore that patients are carefully investigated to rule out other diagnoses.
- Fibromyalgia may occur alongside other conditions, such as rheumatoid arthritis or systemic lupus erythematosus, so it is important to check for markers of rheumatological disease.

CLINICAL FEATURES

- Areas of either widespread or localized tenderness (Fig. 12.1).
- Extreme tiredness and fatigue
- Unrefreshing sleep
- Anxiety
- Depression
- Irritable bowel syndrome
- Muscle stiffness
- Headaches
- Pain which may be dull, sharp or burning in nature
- Patients may have a low tolerance to pain (hyperaesthesia), but they may also suffer pain even with light touch (allodynia).

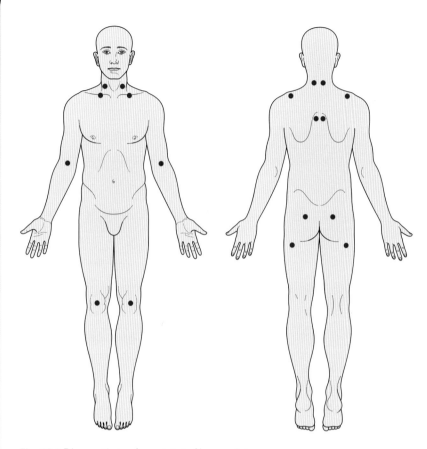

Fig. 12.1 Diagnostic tender points in fibromyalgia.

> ## MICRO-facts
>
> **ACR diagnostic criteria for fibromyalgia**
> Widespread concurrent pain in at least 11 out of 18 defined points on the body for at least three months.

DIAGNOSIS

The American College of Rheumatologists (ACR) devised diagnostic criteria in 1990 primarily for use in clinical trials. Due to the nature of the condition, the diagnosis is often made based on the whole clinical picture, irrespective of whether the criteria are completely met.

In 2010, a further diagnostic aid was devised termed the 'Symptom Severity Score'.

MANAGEMENT

- Lifestyle modification factors, such as exercise, relaxation techniques and improved sleep hygiene.
- Physiotherapy.
- Medication to include analgesia and anti-depressants.
- Cognitive behavioural therapy and psychotherapy.
- Support groups and a good support network can form an important part of a patient's treatment.

13 Spondyloarthritides

13.1 OVERVIEW

- Spondyloarthritides are chronic, multi-system, inflammatory diseases which share a number of characteristics.
- The term 'spondyloarthritides' is used to describe an arthritis with a tendency to involve the spine (hence 'spondylo-').
- While there are several inflammatory joint conditions of this nature, this chapter concentrates on those more commonly encountered in clinical practice. These include:
    - Ankylosing spondylitis (AS)
    - Psoriatic arthritis
    - Reactive arthritis (formerly Reiter's syndrome)
    - Enteropathic arthritis.

The clinical features of spondyloarthritides are described in Table 13.1.

Table 13.1 Clinical features of spondyloarthritides.

MUSCULOSKELETAL	EXTRA-ARTICULAR	GENETIC
Asymmetrical oligoarthritis	Psoriasis	HLA-B27
Sacroiliitis	Iritis	
Spondylitis	Inflammatory bowel disease	
Enthesitis		

HLA-B27

HLA-B27 tissue type has a strong association with spondyloarthritides. It is a risk factor for development any of the spondyloarthritides, particularly ankylosing spondylitis. Note that rheumatoid arthritis is associated with a different histocompatibility antigen, HLA-DR4.

Table 13.2 sets out the prevalence of HLA B27 in the spondyloarthritides.

Table 13.2 Association of HLA-B27 with spondyloarthritides.

CONDITION	% HLA-B27 WITH CONDITION
Ankylosing spondylitis	92
Psoriatic arthritis	60
Reactive arthritis	60
Enteropathic arthritis	60

SACROILITIS

- This may occur in all the spondyloarthritides, but features in all cases of ankylosing spondylitis.
- Buttock pain is the usual presenting feature.
- Early changes are detectable on magnetic resonance image (MRI).
- X-rays show erosion and eventually fusion of the sacroiliac joints in later stage disease.

ASYMMETRY

While rheumatoid arthritis usually affects the joints symmetrically, spondyloarthritides more often than not have an asymmetrical pattern of presentation (Table 13.3).

Table 13.3 Comparison between ankylosing spondylitis and rheumatoid arthritis.

	ANKYLOSING SPONDYLITIS	RHEUMATOID ARTHRITIS
Peak age	Middle age	Middle age
Gender	Male > female (3:1)	Female > male (3:1)
Joint pattern	Oligoarthritis	Polyarthritis
RhF	Always negative	Usually positive
Antigen	HLA-B27	HLA-DR4

OLIGOARTHRITIS

Unlike rheumatoid arthritis which is a polyarthritis, spondyloarthritides affect only a few joints (<5).

ENTHESITIS

The spondyloarthritides target the insertions of tendons and ligaments (entheses) and cause an inflammatory reaction in the local area (enthesitis). Most common sites for this are the Achilles tendon insertion and the plantar fascia.

RHEUMATOID FACTOR-NEGATIVE

Spondyloarthritides are classified as chronic inflammatory arthritides that are negative for IgM rheumatoid factor (RF) (Table 13.4).

Rheumatology

Table 13.4 Extra-articular manifestations of spondyloarthritides.

CONDITION	EXTRA-ARTICULAR MANIFESTATIONS
Ankylosing spondylitis	Aortic valve disease, carditis, pulmonary fibrosis, iritis, amyloidosis
Psoriatic arthritis	Psoriasis
Reactive arthritis	Conjunctivitis, urethritis
Enteropathic arthritis	Enteritis, colitis

FAMILIAL CONTRIBUTION

- Spondyloarthritides often have a familial incidence.
- It is important to take a full family history when admitting a rheumatology patient.
- Close family members may have other features of a spondyloarthritis (i.e. may have psoriasis or iritis even if not arthritis or spondylitis).
- Note the common HLA-B27 tissue type.

MICRO-print
Enthesitis
The tendon/ligament bone attachment site is infiltrated by granulation tissue which comprises leukocytes, plasma cells and lymphocytes. The bone marrow adjacent to the lesion also contains inflammatory cells and excess tissue fluid.

13.2 ANKYLOSING SPONDYLITIS

DEFINITION

- From the Greek *ankylos* meaning 'stiff', *spondylos* meaning 'vertebral disk' and *itis* meaning 'inflammation'.
- The inflammatory process affects the spine and the sacroiliac joints.
- Ankylosing spondylitis is a chronic condition that may persist throughout adult life.
- Sometimes, it may become apparently inactive and symptoms may fluctuate.
- It is rarely 'episodic'.

PREVALANCE

It most commonly first presents in young men between the ages of 20 and 40 years.

CLINICAL FEATURES

- It presents as chronic back pain which radiates into the buttocks, with progressive back stiffness.
- On examination, the patient has reduction in the range of all spinal movement.
- The diagnosis is dependent on recognizing clinical features (e.g. inflammatory back pain, co-morbidities), combined with spinal imaging.
- Magnetic resonance imaging (MRI) is indicated in early disease ('axial spondyloarthritis'); x-rays later.
- When the disease is active, C-reactive protein (CRP) and erythrocyte sedimentation rate (ESR) levels usually, but not always, rise.
- In the later stages, extensive ankylosis may give rise to the x-ray appearance of 'bamboo spine' (see Fig. 13.1).

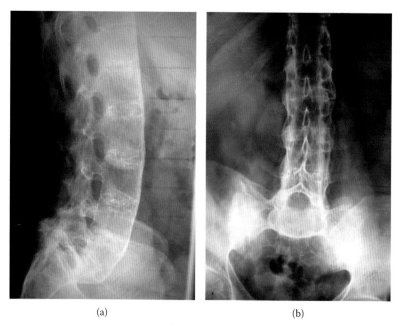

(a)   (b)

Fig. 13.1 Classic bamboo spine appearance seen in ankylosing spondylitis. Reproduced with permission from Williams N, Bulstrode C, O'Connell R. *Bailey & Love's Short Practice of Surgery*, 26th edn. London: Hodder Arnold, 2013.

MICRO-print
Modified Schober's test
- A test of lumbar flexion.
- Mark S1 with a marker pen when patient is erect.

continued...

Rheumatology

continued...

- Make a mark 10 cm above S1 and 5 cm below the S1 using a tape measure.
- Ask patient to bend forward and measure the increase in distance between the marks above and below.
- Normal motion of the lumbar spine should be at least 4–5 cm.

MICRO-reference

van der Linden S, Valkenburg H A, Cats A. Evaluation of diagnostic criteria for ankylosing spondylitis. A proposal for modification of the New York criteria. *Arthritis and Rheumatology* 1984; **27**: 361–8. Available from www.ncbi.nlm.nih.gov/pubmed/6231933

MANAGEMENT

- There is no curative treatment.
- Exercise programmes should be aimed at maintaining upright posture and preventing progressive flexion deformity.
- Physiotherapy.
- Non-steroidal anti-inflammatory drugs (NSAIDs).
- TNF-alpha-blockers, such as infliximab and adalimumab, if the New York criteria are met (as recommended by the National Institute for Health and Clinical Excellence (NICE)) (Table 13.5).

Table 13.5 Modified New York criteria for diagnosing ankylosing spondylitis.

MODIFIED NEW YORK CRITERIA	
Clinical criteria	Low back pain; present for more than three months; improved by exercise but not relieved by rest
	Limitation of lumbar spine motion in both the sagittal and frontal planes
	Limitation of chest expansion relative to normal values for age and sex
Radiological criterion	Sacroiliitis on x-ray
Diagnosis	Definite ankylosing spondylitis if the radiological criterion is present, plus at least one clinical criterion
	Probable ankylosing spondylitis if three clinical criteria are present alone, or if the radiological criterion is present but no clinical criteria are present

Data from van der Linden S, Valkenburg H A, Cats A. Evaluation of diagnostic criteria for ankylosing spondylitis. A proposal for modification of the New York criteria. *Arthritis and Rheumatology* 1984; **27**: 361.

> ### MICRO-case
> Mr. Bridge is a 25-year-old who was recently diagnosed with ankylosing spondylitis. He went to the rheumatology outpatient clinic and told the doctor that his back stiffness and posture were worse and that he was 'tired all the time'. His latest blood results confirmed his ESR was significantly raised and spine x-rays were taken.
>
> ### Points to consider
> - A raised ESR is commonly seen in ankylosing spondylitis.
> - Radiological evidence of ankylosing spondylitis includes sacroiliac sclerosis and new intervertebral syndesmophytes bridging the vertebrae.
> - A late stage lumbar x-ray of ankylosing spondylitis could reveal a 'bamboo spine' (occurs later in the disease process).

SURGERY

Up to a third of patients require hip or knee surgery. Vertebral osteotomy can be performed to improve posture.

13.3 PSORIATIC ARTHRITIS

DEFINITION

Psoriatic arthritis is a spondyloarthritis which is associated with psoriasis.

AETIOLOGY

Psoriatic arthritis has a strong familial preponderance (see Chapter 7, Sacrum and pelvis).

CLINICAL FEATURES

- It usually affects the knees, fingers, ankles and small joints of the hands and feet, causing pain, redness, swelling and joint stiffness.
- Entheseal involvement typically produces heel pain due to either plantar fasciitis or Achilles tendonitis.
- Psoriatic nail changes: onycholysis.

MANAGEMENT

- The management for psoriatic arthritis is two-fold; both the dermatological component and the rheumatological component need to be treated.
- A multidisciplinary approach involving a dermatologist and rheumatologist is required. Management includes:
  - Exercise
  - Topical emollients, steroids and phototherapy for skin lesions

- Anti-inflammatory drug (NSAIDs)
- Disease-modifying anti-rheumatic drugs (DMARDs)
- TNF-α blockers

13.4 REACTIVE ARTHRITIS

DEFINITION

Reactive arthritis is a sterile arthritis associated with either genital-tract or enteric infection. It was formerly known as 'Reiter's disease or syndrome'.

EPIDEMIOLOGY

Reactive arthritis usually affects young men.

CLINICAL FEATURES

- Urogenital reactive arthritis is often associated with:
  - Non-gonococcal urethritis
  - *Chlamydia trachomatis* or *Neisseria gonnorrhoeae* infection.
- Enteric reactive arthritis is usually associated with *Salmonella*, *Campylobacter*, *Shigella* and *Yersinia* bowel infections.
- Reactive arthritis usually affects the large joints, particularly the knee and ankle.
- Due to the acute presentation, it can be confused with other joint diseases, such as acute gout or septic arthritis.
- Extra-articular manifestations include cervicitis, prostatitis, urethritis, diarrhoea and inflammation of the eye including uveitis, conjunctivitis (most common) and episcleritis.

MANAGEMENT

- Genital tract infection should be treated with appropriate antibiotics with tracing and treatment of sexual contacts.
- Enteric infections are usually best allowed to resolve without antimicrobial treatment.
- NSAIDs, DMARDs, oral steroids, local steroid injections (for single joint or enthesis sites), may be used to treat reactive arthritis.
- Most patients recover completely, but some develop chronic arthritis or AS.

MICRO-print

A sentence to remember the clinical picture of urogenital reactive arthritis: 'Can't see, can't pee, can't climb up a tree':
- Conjunctivitis
- Urethritis
- Arthritis.

MICRO-case

Private Smith is a 19-year-old soldier who has just returned from an overseas tour of duty. He presents to the regimental doctor with persistent pain in his left knee that has come on over 3 weeks. On examination, his knee is hot, red, tender and swollen. He also mentions that he has an 'itchy eye' and has 'a bit of soreness down below when I pass water'. A probable diagnosis of reactive arthritis is made.

Points to consider

- The patient has a reactive arthritis caused by a urogenital infection.
- He requires a full sexual health screen, as well as an x-ray of the knee and routine blood tests such as full blood count (FBC), urea and electrolytes (U&E) and liver function tests (LFT).
- Supportive treatment should be given for the knee symptoms while the infection is treated with the appropriate antibiotics.

13.5 ENTEROPATHIC ARTHRITIS

DEFINITION

Enteropathic arthritis is associated with chronic inflammatory bowel disease, particularly Crohn's disease and ulcerative colitis (UC).

AETIOLOGY

The causal link between irritable bowel disease (IBD) and arthritis has not been proven, but is postulated to be due to leakiness of the bowel mucosa and subsequent exposure to arthritis-provoking antigens.

CLINICAL FEATURES

- Enteropathic arthritis usually affects the large joints, particularly the knee and ankle, often with sacroiliitis, but may resemble rheumatoid arthritis.
- The differential diagnosis includes other acute arthritides, such as acute gout or septic arthritis, and rheumatoid arthritis or other spondyloarthritides. Extra-articular manifestations include enthesitis and uveitis.

MANAGEMENT

- Sulfasalazine is often used in enteropathic arthritis, as it may additionally improve the bowel disease.
- Monoarthritic disease may be treated with intra-articular steroids.
- NSAIDs may improve symptoms, but risk aggravating IBD. They must be used with caution, if at all.
- Anti-TNFα agents are used in Crohn's disease (not in UC) and may also improve the joint symptoms.

14 Vasculitides

14.1 INTRODUCTION TO VASCULITIS

DEFINITION

- Vasculitis is defined by inflammation of blood vessels anywhere in the body.

AETIOLOGY

Primary autoimmune

- Large vessel:
  - Giant cell (temporal) arteritis (GCA)
  - Takayasu arteritis
- Medium vessel:
  - Polyarteritis nodosa (PAN)
  - Kawasaki's disease
- Small ± medium vessel:
  - Microscopic polyangiitis
  - Wegener's granulomatosis
  - Churg–Strauss syndrome
  - Goodpasture syndrome
  - Vasculitis from connective tissue diseases, e.g. systemic lupus erythromatosus (SLE), rheumatoid arthritis (RA), Sjögren's syndrome
  - Henoch–Schönlein purpura (HSP)
  - Behçet syndrome.

Secondary autoimmune

- To infection: e.g. in HIV, syphilis.
- To drugs: e.g. antibiotics, thiazide diuretics, non-inflammatory auto-immune drugs (NSAIDs), etc.
- To malignancy.

CLINICAL FEATURES

- These are legion, given that any blood vessel may be affected (Fig. 14.1).
- Particular features are more common in different conditions, see below under Investigations.

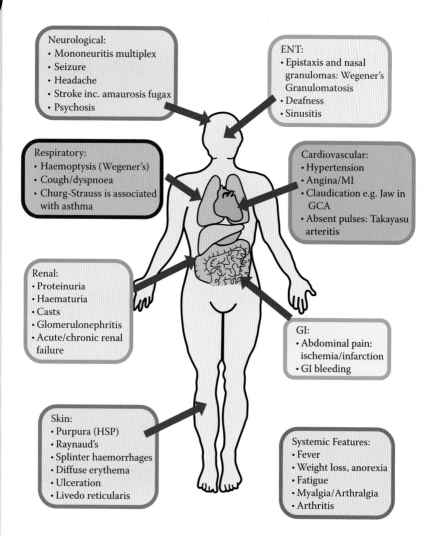

Neurological:
- Mononeuritis multiplex
- Seizure
- Headache
- Stroke inc. amaurosis fugax
- Psychosis

ENT:
- Epistaxis and nasal granulomas: Wegener's Granulomatosis
- Deafness
- Sinusitis

Respiratory:
- Haemoptysis (Wegener's)
- Cough/dyspnoea
- Churg-Strauss is associated with asthma

Cardiovascular:
- Hypertension
- Angina/MI
- Claudication e.g. Jaw in GCA
- Absent pulses: Takayasu arteritis

Renal:
- Proteinuria
- Haematuria
- Casts
- Glomerulonephritis
- Acute/chronic renal failure

GI:
- Abdominal pain: ischemia/infarction
- GI bleeding

Skin:
- Purpura (HSP)
- Raynaud's
- Splinter haemorrhages
- Diffuse erythema
- Ulceration
- Livedo reticularis

Systemic Features:
- Fever
- Weight loss, anorexia
- Fatigue
- Myalgia/Arthralgia
- Arthritis

Fig 14.1 Clinical features of vasculitides.

INVESTIGATIONS

- Inflammatory markers
  - White cell count (WCC)
  - C-reactive protein (CRP), erythrocyte sedimentation rate (ESR)
- Anti-neutrophil cytoplasmic antibodies (ANCA)
  - Anti-PR3: Aka cANCA (cytoplasmic)
    - Wegener's granulomatosis: 80% are positive
    - Microscopic polyangiitis (less commonly than pANCA)
    - Churg–Strauss (less commonly than pANCA).

- Anti-MPO: or pANCA (perinuclear)
  - Churg–Strauss: 60% positive
  - Microscopic polyangiitis (more commonly than cANCA)
  - Wegener's granulomatosis 15% are positive
- Rheumatoid factor
  - May be positive in many vasculitides
  - May indicate RA as a cause.
- Anti-nuclear antibody titre (ANA)
  - Overall ANA titre may be high in vasculitis.
- Specific antibody tests including: anti-double-stranded DNA (anti-dsDNA).
  - Highly specific for SLE: anti-Smith (anti-Sm).
    - SLE: anti-Ro (anti-SSA), anti-La (anti SSB).
  - Sjögren's syndrome.
- Biopsy may provide definitive diagnosis if taken from relevant site, e.g. temporal artery in GCA, renal if kidney involvement.
- Angiography may be useful, e.g. in microscopic polyangiitis, Takayasu's and PAN.
- Urea and electrolytes are undertaken to assess renal involvement.
- Urinalysis for haematuria, casts and proteinuria in glomerulonephritis.

TREATMENT

- Steroids
- Cyclophosphamide or other immune suppression
- Plasma exchange or intravenous immunoglobulin in severe cases.

14.2 GIANT CELL ARTERITIS (TEMPORAL ARTERITIS)

EPIDEMIOLOGY

- Associated with increased age.
- Very uncommon in patients <55 years.
- Associated with polymyalgia rheumatica (PMR) in 25–50% of cases (see below under 14.3 Polymyalgia rheumatica).

CLINICAL FEATURES

Clinical features include:
- Headache, usually temporal
  - Aggravated by combing hair on the affected side
- Jaw claudication
  - Claudication causing pain on mastication
- Amaurosis fugax
  - Central retinal artery ischemia

- Classically presents as 'a curtain falling in front of vision' with visual loss proceeding inferiorly
  - May present as sudden monocular painless visual loss.
- General systemic features (see Fig. 14.1).
- Anti-nuclear antibody titre (ANA)
  - Overall ANA titre may be high in vasculitis.

MANAGEMENT

- Start high-dose steroids, e.g. prednisolone 40–60 mg immediately. Do not wait for test results, medication can be stopped if proven negative. Response is usually quick and within 24–48 hours.
- Contact ophthalmology urgently in cases of visual disturbance.
- If diagnosis confirmed, steroids may be continued for ~2 years.

MICRO-facts

Giant cell arteritis is a medical emergency:
- It may lead to visual loss.
- If suspected, perform an ESR.
- Start high dose steroids immediately.

14.3 POLYMYALGIA RHEUMATICA

DEFINITION

- Inflammatory disorder affecting proximal muscle groups in older adults.
- Not actually a vasculitis, but mentioned here because of its association with GCA, occuring in up to 20% of patients with PMR.

CLINICAL FEATURES

- More common in females 3:1
- More common as age increases
- Very rare <50
- Pain in the shoulder girdle, pelvic muscles
- Systemic features – see Fig. 14.1.

MANAGEMENT

- ESR is usually >60, CRP is elevated, creatine kinase (CK) is usually normal.
- Liver function tests (LFTs) may be deranged (alkaline phosphatase (ALP)/ gamma-glutamyl transpeptidase (GGT)).
- Steroid therapy, e.g. prednisolone 15 mg daily, should be reduced over time. Treat for 1–1.5 years. Patient may need maintenance doses. The response is usually rapid. Watch for signs of GCA.

> **MICRO-print**
> Takayasu arteritis: also known as 'pulseless disease':
> - Vasculitis affecting the aorta and key branches.
> - Leads to absent pulses and claudication pain in arms, with systemic features.
> - Treatment is with steroids after angiographic diagnosis.

14.4 WEGENER'S GRANULOMATOSIS

DEFINITION

- Granulomatous vasculitis affects medium to small vessels
- Rare: incidence of ~4 per million

CLINICAL FEATURES

- Systemic features Fig. 14.1. They commonly affect the upper respiratory tract, including epistaxis and granulomas.
- Pulmonary granulomas and haemorrhages
  - Haemoptysis
  - Medical emergency.
- Renal involvement includes glomerulonephritis.
- Skin, eye and joint involvement is also common.

MANAGEMENT

- cANCA elevated (see above under Investigations)
- Urinalysis (see above under Investigations)
- Chest x-ray for pulmonary haemorrhage
- Cyclophosphamide and steroids ± plasma exchange in pulmonary haemorrhage (seek specialist input).
- Renal specialist input for management of glomerulonephritis e.g. steroids.

14.5 CHURG–STRAUSS SYNDROME

DEFINITION

Churg-Strauss syndrome is a rare multisystem vasculitis associated with asthma.

CLINICAL FEATURES AND MANAGEMENT

- Patients typically have a long-standing history of asthma.
- pANCA is elevated (see above under Investigations).
- Eosinophilia ± eosinophilic pneumonia.
- Renal involvement includes glomerulonephritis.
- Mononeuritis multiplex.
- Systemic features (see Fig. 14.1).
- Treatment is with steroids ± immunosuppression: seek specialist involvement.

14.6 POLYARTERITIS NODOSA

DEFINITION

Polyarteritis nodosa (PAN) is a rare multisystem vasculitis of medium-sized vessels with microaneurysm formation.

CLINICAL FEATURES AND MANAGEMENT

- Systemic features (see Fig. 14.1).
- Gastrointestinal (GI) involvement: mesenteric artery vasculitis with abdominal pain.
- Renal involvement is common and includes glomerulonephritis.
- Cardiovascular vasculitis including of coronary arteries.
- Neurological (see Fig. 14.1).
- Skin involvement.
- Associated with hepatitis B infection.
- ANCA usually negative.
- Treatment is with steroids or immunosuppression.

14.7 MICROSCOPIC POLYANGIITIS

DEFINITION

Microscopic polyangiitis is a rare multisystem vasculitis largely affecting the small vessels.

CLINICAL FEATURES AND MANAGEMENT

- pANCA is usually positive; cANCA may be positive less commonly.
- Renal involvement including glomerulonephritis.
- Lungs: haemoptysis/haemorrhage.
- Skin: purpura.
- Similar to Wegener's granulomatosis (note pANCA predominates here).
- As with other vasculitides, may present anywhere (see Fig. 14.1).

MICRO-print
Kawasaki's disease

- Small vessel vasculitis affecting children usually <5 years
- Mucocutaneous bleeding
- 'Five day fever', then thrombocytosis and rash
- Cardiovascular features: coronary aneurysms and myocardial infarction (MI)
- Lymphadenopathy
- Treatment with intravenous immunoglobulin

Behçet syndrome

- Rare vasculitis affecting arteries and venules
- Recurrent oral and genital ulceration
- Anterior uveitis
- Pathergy is pathognomonic: pustules form at site of skin injury, e.g. venepuncture
- Other features of systemic vasculitis (see Fig. 14.1)

14.8 GOODPASTURE SYNDROME

DEFINITION

Goodpasture syndrome is a rare autoimmune condition with autoantibodies against glomerular basement membranes (anti-GBM) affecting capillary beds in lungs and kidneys.

CLINICAL FEATURES AND MANAGEMENT

- Anti-GBM positive
- Pulmonary haemorrhage and haemoptysis: investigate with chest x-ray
- Haematuria and glomerulonephritis: investigate with renal biopsy
- Note absence of symptoms outside these two areas given specific antibody target.
- Treatment is with immunosupresssion, steroids and plasma exchange.

15 Crystal arthropathies

15.1 GOUT

DEFINITION

Gout is a very painful, rapidly accelerating monoarthritis caused by deposition of monosodium urate crystals in a joint.

EPIDEMIOLOGY

- Male > female
- Most common cause of monoarthritis in men aged 40–60 years and occurs in women after the menopause or secondary to other pathologies.

AETIOLOGY

- There is a causal link between increasing hyperuricaemia and gout, however, serum uric acid levels may be low or normal in acute attack.
- There are several aetiological risk factors for developing gout:
  - Age: older > younger
  - Body size: large > small
  - Socioeconomic status: high > low

PATHOPHYSIOLOGY

- Purines and hyperuricaemia
  - Gout is a consequence of the lack of the enzyme uricase in humans.
  - In other mammals, this oxidizes urate into the easily soluble allantoin.
  - When purines (derived from nucleic acids) are metabolized, they are broken down to uric acid. Most uric acid is excreted by the kidneys, although about a third is excreted by the gut.
  - Not all people with hyperuricaemia will develop gout. However, acute gouty arthritis results from saturation of tissues by uric acid with deposition of monosodium urate crystals.
  - Gout may also be precipitated by an injury or knock to the joint or by dehydration.

CLINICAL FEATURES

- Symptoms peak after 6–12 hours.
- Hot, painful, swollen, tender joint.
- Most commonly affects the first metatarsophalangeal joint (podagra), although may affect the knee, mid-tarsal joints, wrists, ankles, elbows and small joints of the hand (Fig. 15.1).
- May be associated with chronic renal damage.
- Low-grade fever, general malaise and anorexia.

RISK FACTORS FOR GOUT

- Risk factors linked with under-excretion of urate include:
  - Renal impairment
  - Hypertension
  - Drugs: thiazide diuretics and low-dose aspirin
  - Type II diabetes mellitus
  - Hypothyroidism
  - Hyperparathyroidism.

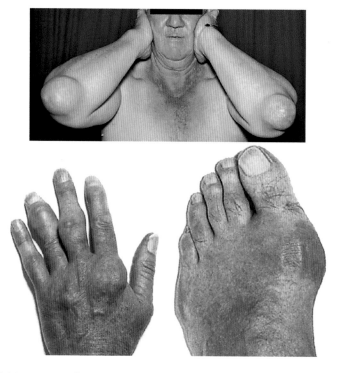

Fig. 15.1 Acute gout, showing redness, swelling and scaling of overlying skin. Reproduced with permission from Solomon L, Warwick D, Nayagam S (eds.). *Apley's System of Orthopaedics and Fractures*, 9th edn. London: Hodder Arnold, 2010.

Rheumatology

MICRO-facts

- Decreased urate excretion
  - Renal failure
- Increased urate production
  - Haematological disorders, such as lymphoproliferative and myeloproliferative disorders e.g. polycythaemia
  - Haemolytic anaemia
  - Severe psoriasis
  - Carcinomatosis
  - Cytotoxic chemotherapy: high turnover of cells
- Inborn error in purine metabolism
  - Genetic enzyme defects
- Increased purine intake
  - Increased intake of beer, red meat and dietary fructose.

Please note: dehydration after an alcoholic binge is more likely to be responsible for an attack than the beer consumption itself!

POLYARTICULAR GOUT

- More common in elderly patients.
- Polyarticular gout usually affects joints on only one side of the patient's body.
- The onset of pain is slower than in acute gout and it may take 24–48 hours before maximal pain.
- Usually affects joints in the extremities: hands and feet.

MICRO-print

It is thought that polyarticular gout usually affects joints in the hands and feet due to crystallization of urate crystals occurring more readily at lower temperatures.

PRIMARY AND SECONDARY GOUT

- Primary:
  - Enzyme deficiencies
  - Undersecretion of uric acid.
- Secondary to an identifiable cause, including:
  - Metabolic disturbances
  - Drugs (e.g. thiazide diuretics)
  - Renal injury or acquired impairment.

MICRO-print

Gout rarely occurs in children, but if seen, inherited deficiency of the enzyme hypoxanthine guanine phosphoribosyl transferase (HGPRT) should be considered. Complete absence of this enzyme is seen in Lesch–Nyhan syndrome.

MICRO-facts

It is important to identify any underlying causative factors that can be removed to aid treatment and reduce risk of recurrence:
- In the elderly, it is most likely to be drug induced. Ask about thiazide diuretics and aspirin usage.
- In the younger population, careful investigation is required to determine the cause.

DIAGNOSIS

- Diagnosis is usually clinical, however, the gold standard for diagnosing gout is joint aspiration of synovial fluid.
- Urate crystals can be seen with a microscope under polarized light. They are needle-shaped and strongly negatively birefringent (Fig. 15.2).

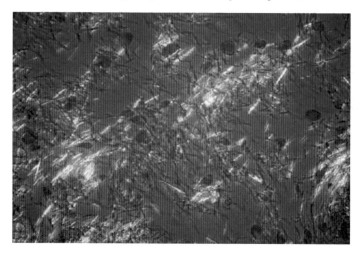

Fig. 15.2 Negatively birefringent crystals as seen in gout. Reproduced with permission from Solomon L, Warwick D, Nayagam S (eds.). *Apley's System of Orthopaedics and Fractures*, 9th edn. London: Hodder Arnold, 2010.

INVESTIGATIONS

Examination
- Synovial fluid by polarized light microscopy for urate crystals
- Blood pressure.

Blood tests
- Plasma urate level
- Renal function
- Cholesterol
- Blood glucose
- Thyroid function (15% of patients with gout have hypothyroidism)
- Liver enzymes: possible alcohol abuse.
- Care must be taken when interpreting plasma urate levels in an acute attack as serum levels may actually decrease.
- Conversely, evidence of hyperuricaemia on blood tests does not mean a patient has or will have gout.
- Plasma urate levels are useful in monitoring the response to therapy, such as before and after treatment with allopurinol.
- X-rays of the affected joint are not useful in the diagnosis of acute gout as only soft tissue swelling will be seen.
- In the patient who has had long-standing recurrent gout, then it is likely that erosions with overhanging edges will be seen with surrounding sclerotic bone.

MANAGEMENT
- High-dose non-steroidal anti-inflammatory drugs (NSAIDs) (usually co-prescribed with a proton pump inhibitor (PPI)).
- Colchicine either twice or three times a day (if more frequent, then likely to cause severe diarrhoea).
- Corticosteroids (either systemic or as an intra-articular injection) are particularly useful if the patient cannot tolerate taking either NSAIDs or colchicine.

MICRO-facts
It is important to send a sample of the aspirate for Gram staining and cultures as it is vital that an infected joint is not missed.

Rheumatology

MICRO-case

Mr Sellens is a 63-year-old male with polycystic kidney disease. He has severely impaired renal function and requires haemodialysis three times per week. This patient presents to the hospital with a 1-day history of an acutely inflamed, very tender first MTP (metatarsophalangeal) joint that woke him from his sleep. He has a low-grade fever. Serum urate levels and x-ray are normal.

The most likely diagnosis in this case is acute gout and so you start the patient on NSAIDs with PPI cover and colchicine.

Points to consider

- To make a firm diagnosis, a joint aspirate is required and viewed under microscopy with polarized light.
- Negatively birefringenet, needle-shaped crystals are seen under microscopy.
- Plasma urate levels may actually decrease in acute gout.
- In acute gout, x-rays are only likely to show soft tissue inflammation so are of little benefit.

CHRONIC GOUT

Chronic gout occurs due to years of recurrent acute gout attacks with uncontrolled hyperuricaemia. It is characterized by:

- Development of tophi (monosodium urate crystal deposits) around the ears, hands, elbows and feet.
- Joint destruction: erosions with overhanging edges may be seen on radiographs.

COMPLICATIONS

- Nephropathy occurs due to deposition of urate crystals in the renal interstitium causing inflammation and fibrosis.
- Urate stones also may develop in the urinary tract of patients with gout and therefore serum urate should be measured in patients with renal colic.

MICRO-facts

The development of tophi and chronic gout can contribute to a destructive arthropathy and osteoarthritis.

TREATMENT

- Symptomatic chronic gouty joints require similar treatment to acute episodes as above. In this situation, reduction of the urate load is also crucial; a xanthine oxidase inhibitor (usually allopurinol) is appropriate.
- As allopurinol is excreted via the kidneys, dose adjustments must be made in renal impairment.

PROPHYLAXIS

Patients with asymptomatic hyperuricaemia and normal kidney function do not require treatment.

Indications for prophylaxis

- Recurrent attacks (two or more per year).
- The presence of tophi.
- Polyarticular disease.
- Renal disease/impairment.

Prophylactic treatment

- Reduction of urate load by xanthine oxidase inhibitor (usually allopurinol, but febuxostat may also be used).
- Regular NSAIDs or colchicine to reduce the likelihood and severity of acute attacks after initiation of xanthine-oxidase inhibitor therapy.

MICRO-facts

Allopurinol must not be started for at least 1–2 weeks after the acute gout attack.

Changes in serum urate can either delay a resolution of symptoms or precipitate an acute attack of gout. To reduce the risk of this, colchicine and NSAIDs should also be prescribed for the first 6–18 months.

MICRO-case

A 70-year-old woman presents to her GP complaining of raised lumps on her knuckles and ears. She is known to have a past history of recurrent gout, stretching back over ten years. You recognize these lumps as being typical of gouty tophi. They are caused by crystal deposits in the tissues.

Points to consider

- Gouty tophi may remain the same, increase in size or resolve with urate-lowering therapy.
- Tophi are pathognomonic for gout.
- Thiazide diuretics and aspirin have both been shown to increase the likelihood of developing tophaceous gout.

15.2 PSEUDOGOUT

DEFINITION

- Pseudogout, as the name suggests, may be easily confused with gout. However, instead of urate, pseudogout is an acute monoarthritis caused by the deposition of calcium pyrophosphate dihydrate (CPPD) crystals.

- It has been shown to be associated with the following conditions:
  - Hypothyroidism
  - Hypercalcaemia
  - Hypomagnesaemia
  - Haemochromatosis.
- The most commonly affected site is the knee, however, the following joints may also be affected:
  - Shoulder
  - Hand
  - Wrist
  - Elbow.

PRESENTATION

Similar to gout, but usually milder, pseudogout is characterized by an acute mono- or oligo-arthritis that has:
- Swelling
- Effusion
- Warmth
- Tenderness
- Pain on movement.

DIAGNOSIS

Aspiration of the affected joint yields synovial fluid that contains rhomboid crystals that are weakly positively birefringent when viewed by polarized light microscopy (Fig. 15.3).

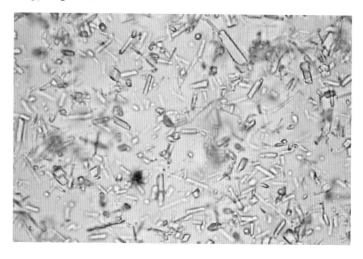

Fig. 15.3 Weakly positively birefringent crystals as seen in pseudogout. Reproduced with permission from Solomon L, Warwick D, Nayagam S (eds.). *Apley's System of Orthopaedics and Fractures*, 9th edn. London: Hodder Arnold, 2010.

MICRO-facts

It is important to send a sample of the aspirate for Gram staining and cultures as it is vital that an infected joint is not missed.
X-ray of the affected joint may show:
- Chondrocalcinosis (often seen in the menisci of the knee, triangular cartilage of the wrist and the symphysis pubis)
- Changes of osteoarthritis.

TREATMENT OPTIONS OF ACUTE PSEUDOGOUT

- Intra-articular steroid joint injection
- Colchicine
- NSAIDs.

TREATMENT OPTIONS FOR CHRONIC PSEUDOGOUT

There are no specific treatments available, but the following may improve symptoms and help prevent recurrence:
- NSAIDs
- Colchicine
- Treatment of associated osteoarthritis, including:
    - Weight reduction
    - Physiotherapy.

MICRO-case

A 60-year-old male presents to Accident and Emergency with a painful swollen right knee, but denies any history of trauma or previous episodes. On x-ray, articular chondrocalcinosis is seen. You therefore make a provisional diagnosis of pseudogout, but know you need to obtain a joint aspirate to confirm your diagnosis and to rule out intra-articular infection.

After obtaining the results, you give the gentleman an intra-articular steroid injection and start him on ibuprofen with a PPI cover.

Points to consider
- In pseudogout, the synovial fluid contains rhomboid crystals that are weakly positively birefringent when viewed by polarized light microscopy.
- Before taking a joint aspirate, it is vital that you ensure the patient does not have a joint replacement. If so, orthopaedics must be contacted.
- Intra-articular steroid joint injection, colchicine and NSAIDs are all treatment options in acute episodes.

16 Non-inflammatory arthroses

16.1 OSTEOARTHRITIS

DEFINITION

- Osteoarthritis (OA) is a common, chronic, non-inflammatory disease of non-synovial and synovial joints.
- It is characterized by loss of cartilage and subsequent bone remodelling.
- Recent research confirms that the condition is a metabolically reactive, reparative process.

EPIDEMIOLOGY

- Affects over 80% of the population of the Western World at some point in their life.
- The majority are asymptomatic.
- It is rare in those < 45 years old.
- Incidence increases with age.
- Female > males, especially in hand and knee joints.
- More common in Caucasians.

> **MICRO-print**
> OA is thought to select certain joints that have gone through recent evolutionary change (hip and knee because of bipedal locomotion). Primary nodal OA seems to have specific genetic links, so joint distribution may be genetically determined in part.

RISK FACTORS

Modifiable

The listed risk factors are all inter-related in causation:
- Obesity
    - Change in lifestyle and diet is responsible for the obesity epidemic in Western society.
    - Increase in body mass index (BMI) adds to joint load with secondary 'wear and tear'.

- Occupation
  - The type of work undertaken by the western population (the shift from more active manual to sedentary work) adds to the risk of OA.
- Exercise
  - Sedentary lifestyle coupled with long working hours results in less time for exercise.
  - However, excessive use (for example, seen in plasterers' shoulders) and injuries sustained contributes to early onset OA.

Non-modifiable

- Age
- Joint malalignment
- Genetic predisposition
- Gender
- Trauma, e.g. meniscus or cruciate injury.

PATHOGENESIS

- OA is not regarded as a simple 'wear and tear' degenerative process affecting synovial joints, but is an active metabolic disease process resulting in net joint cartilage degradation.
- The acronym 'LOSS' is useful in remembering the pathology, as well as the x-ray features of OA (Fig. 16.1).

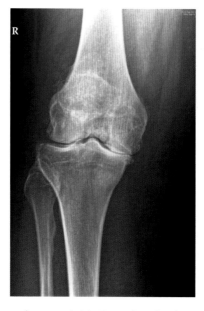

Fig. 16.1 X-ray features of osteoarthritis. Reproduced with permission from Black J, Burnand K, Thomas W et al. (eds.). *Browse's Introduction to the Investigation and Management of Surgical Disease*. London: Hodder Arnold, 2010.

Rheumatology

- Loss of joint space
- Osteophytes
- Subcrondral cysts
- Sclerosis.
- Late-stage OA may show features, such as:
    - Ulceration of cartilage
    - Synovial inflammation.

CLINICAL FEATURES

- Unlike rheumatoid arthritis (RA), there are no extra-articular features of OA (Tables 16.1 and 16.2).
- Any joint can be affected, most commonly, hip, knee, thumb carpo-metacarpal joint (Fig. 16.2), distal interphalangeal (DIP) joint, proximal interphalangeal (PIP), cervical and lumbar spine.
- Classical features are joint stiffness, swelling and deformity of gradual onset over many years.
- Typically monoarthritic joint disease.
    - However, primary nodal (DIP joint) OA is very common and is polyarticular.
    - Pain, stiffness and bony swelling of the involved joints.

Table 16.1 Combined clinical (history, physical examination, laboratory) and radiographic classification criteria for osteoarthritis of the hip.

1	Hip pain *and*
2	Femoral and/or acetabular osteophytes on radiograph *or*
3a	ESR ≤20 mm/hour *and*
3b	Axial joint space narrowing on radiograph

This classification method yields a sensitivity of 91% and a specificity of 89%.

ESR, ethryocyte sedimentation rate (Webstergren).

Reproduced with permission from Altman R, Alarcón G, Appelrouth D *et al*. The American College of Rheumatology criteria for the classification and reporting of osteoarthritis of the hip. *Arthritis and Rheumatism* 1991; 34: 505–14.

Table 16.2 Classification of osteoarthritis of the knee.

Knee pain plus osteophytes on radiographs and at least one of the following:
Patient age older than 50 years
Morning stiffness lasting 30 minutes or less
Crepitus on motion

Reproduced with permission from Altman R, Asch E, Bloch D *et al*. Development of criteria for the classification and reporting of osteoarthritis: classification of osteoarthritis of the knee. *Arthritis and Rheumatism* 1986; 29: 1039–49.

Rheumatology

(a)

(b)

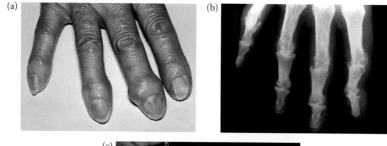

(c)

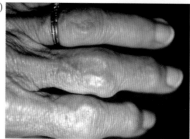

Fig. 16.2 Osteoarthritic changes of the hand (a–c). Reproduced with permission from Solomon L, Warwick D, Nayagam S (eds). *Apley's System of Orthopaedics and Fractures*, 9th edn. London: Hodder Arnold, 2010.

- Increasing difficulty with activities of daily living, such as getting dressed.
- Stiffness increases the more the joint is used.
- Pain increases with activity.
- At the end of the day, stiffness is more common and sleep is disturbed by joint pain.

MICRO-facts

Some specific joint changes that are useful to remember:
- Baker's cyst: an effusion in the posterior knee secondary to knee OA, but also any persistent knee synovitis including RA
- Heberden's node: distal interpharyngeal joint (DIP) OA
- Bouchard's node: proximal interpharyngeal joint (PIP) OA.

MICRO-print

Baker's (popliteal) cyst can present as popliteal vein compression giving the clinical signs of a deep vein thrombosis (DVT). This is known as pseudo-thrombophlebitis (PTP).

Rheumatology

TYPES OF OA

Large joint

- Typically knee or hip
- Knee OA can include medial femorotibial, lateral tibiofemoral or patellofemoral involvement. Medial femorotibial is likely to cause the greatest degree of disability.
- Knee OA is closely associated with obesity.
- Hip OA with superolateral displacement of the femoral head is most likely to progress to a stage requiring surgery.

Primary

- Nodal OA
  - Female > male.
  - Polyarticular, mainly in the hands.
  - Heberden's and Bouchard's nodes commonly present.
  - Disease often favours more distal joints, with proximal hand and the wrist joints being spared.
- Erosive OA
  - Much rarer than nodal OA and is inflammatory.
  - Commonly affects the hands with distal and proximal interphalangeal joints affected with similar severity.
  - More likely to cause disability than nodal OA as the joints are much more unstable.

Secondary

- OA is seen secondary to many different pathologies.
- Some of the more common are:
  - Metabolic:
    - Gout
    - Haemachromatosis
    - Wilson's disease
    - Acromegaly
    - Hyperparathyroidism.
  - Neuropathic:
    - Diabetes mellitus.

INVESTIGATIONS

Bloods tests

- None specific to OA.
- Full blood count (FBC), C-reactive protein (CRP), erythrocyte sedimentation rate (ESR), plasma viscosity, rheumatoid factor, anti-cyclic citrullinated peptide (anti-CCP), auto-antibodies to exclude other rheumatological conditions.

Imaging

- X-rays of affected joints are the mainstay of diagnosis.
- Magnetic resonance imaging (MRI) or ultrasound imaging of the joint, if effusion is present or for differential diagnosis.

Aspiration of synovial fluid

Aspiration of synovial fluid is rarely performed unless diagnosis is uncertain and presentation is atypical.

MICRO-case

Frank Creasy is a 62-year-old man who presents with left knee pain at the orthopaedic outpatients' clinic. He complains of a long-standing progressively severe pain in his left knee that is worse after strenuous activity. On examination, you find the knee has marked crepitus on flexion. He is otherwise fit and has an active lifestyle. He is worried because the pain is starting to make a significant impact on his work and social activities. You arrange x-rays, on the basis of which you diagnose knee OA.

Points to consider

Four changes that are likely to be present on his radiographs (LOSS: loss of joint space, osteophytes, subchrondral cysts and sclerosis).

DIFFERENTIAL DIAGNOSIS

- Pseudogout
- Gout
- Referred pain
- Bursitis
- Psoriatic arthritis
- Spondyloarthritis
- Rheumatoid arthritis.

MANAGEMENT

- Modifiable risks factors are given above under Risk factors. They should be addressed in all OA patients.
- Exercise must be recommended regardless of severity of OA. This aids:
  - Weight loss
  - Improvement in general fitness
  - Increasing muscle bulk around the affected joint
  - Pain control
  - Maintenance of joint function.
- Current guidance advises a holistic approach to OA: lifestyle, education and exercise are all important for successful management.
- Non-pharmaceutical intervention is an important component in the management of OA and should be discussed with the patient before moving on to medical and surgical management.

Rheumatology

> **MICRO-reference**
>
> National Institute for Health and Clinical Excellence. Osteoarthritis.
> Available from: www.nice.org.uk/Search.do?searchText =
> osteoarthritis&newsearch = true&x = 0&y = 0#/search/?reload

---

MICRO-facts

The holistic approach to managing OA

The following treatments are recommended in the current National Institute for Health and Clinical Excellence (NICE) guidance:
- Thermotherapy: hot and cold packs
- Capsaicin cream
- Transcutaneous electrical nerve stimulation (TENS)
- Foot supports and braces
- Occupational therapy
- Physiotherapy

Pharmacological interventions

A 'stepwise' approach is recommended:
- Simple analgesics: start with paracetamol.
- Non-steroidal anti-inflammatory drugs (NSAIDs): combine pain relief and decrease joint inflammation. Start with topical before oral NSAIDs as side effects are less likely.
- Steroids: given by intra-articular injection, the beneficial effects last from 3 to 4 weeks up to six months.

MICRO-print

Always discuss the side effects of intra-articular steroid treatment with the patient:
- Tendon weakness
- Skin changes (pigmentation and atrophy)
- Infection (very rare)
- Intra-articular injections should be limited to a maximum of three per year.

Surgical intervention

Refer the patient to an orthopaedic surgeon if symptoms persist after non-surgical interventions have been tried and symptoms make a significant impact on the patient's quality of life.

- Arthroscopy: there is no supportive evidence of benefit, unless there are loose bodies within the joint that affect movement and are causing secondary joint swelling.
- Joint replacement ± resurfacing: offers pain relief, improves function and overall quality of life. Hip and knee joints are the most common joints to be replaced in OA.

16.2 OSTEONECROSIS

DEFINITION

Osteonecrosis is defined as death of bone due to inadequate or disrupted blood supply.

EPIDEMIOLOGY

- The disease is more common in men and usually presents between the ages of 20 and 50 years old, although it can happen at any age.
- Osteonecrosis can occur in any joint, but it most commonly occurs in the femoral head, the lunate, the waist of the scaphoid and neck of the talus

AETIOLOGY/PATHOPHYSIOLOGY

- Osteonecrosis can be caused by several different mechanisms.
- It can be caused by a break in the bone or dislocation.
- Many risk factors are associated with the disease, such as steroids, radiation therapy, alcohol, sickle cell disease, systemic lupus erythematosis and bisphosphonates.
- High-dose bisphosphonates (as used in the treatment of certain cancers) are well known to be a leading cause of osteonecrosis of the jaw.
- The blood supply to the bone is disrupted leading to under-perfusion and cell death.
- It should be noted that osteonecrosis of the femoral head in children is known as Legg–Calvé–Perthes syndrome.

CLINICAL FEATURES

- There may be a history of trauma which resulted in a fracture of the bone or dislocation of a joint.
- The patient may not complain of pain until marked necrosis has occurred.
- Make sure that a thorough history is taken to ensure that any risk factors for osteonecrosis that the patient may have are identified.

EXAMINATION

The patient will have a decreased range of movement and there will be pain on movement of the affected joint.

Rheumatology

INVESTIGATIONS

- Bone scintigraphy
- MRI
- X-rays

MANAGEMENT

- Treatment depends on the joint involved.
- Osteonecrosis in the hip is commonly treated by performing a total hip replacement, and joint replacements can be performed at other sites.
- Osteotomy can be utilized in the management of the disease.
- Core decompression is also sometimes used, where part of the core of the bone is taken out, thus decompressing that area of bone so that new blood vessel formation is stimulated.
- Bone grafts can also be performed.
- Adequate analgesia will need to be prescribed.

17 Disorders of bone metabolism

17.1 OSTEOPOROSIS

DEFINITION

- Osteoporosis is a systemic skeletal disease characterized by low bone mass and microarchitectural deterioration of bone tissue. This results in an increase in bone fragility and likelihood of sustaining a fracture.
- It is defined as a T-score of less than or equal to 2.5 SD (standard deviations) below the young adult reference mean score at the lumbar spine or hip.

> **MICRO-facts**
>
> As there are no symptoms and the first presentation is often a fracture, it is known as the 'silent disease'.

- Many students confuse osteoporosis with osteomalacia and although many effects of the two diseases overlap, they are very different conditions. Osteomalacia is covered in detail below under 17.3 Osteomalacia.

EPIDEMIOLOGY

- It is very common metabolic bone disorder.
- There is increasing incidence with aging population.
- Almost three million people in the UK are estimated to have osteoporosis.
- Fifty per cent of women and 20% of men over the age of 50 will have an osteoporotic fracture in their remaining lifetime.

PATHOPHYSIOLOGY

- Bone undergoes constant remodelling in the adult skeleton with osteoclastic bone resorption and osteoblastic bone formation occurring all the time in discrete bone remodelling units.
- The human skeleton consists of approximately 20% trabecular bone and 80% cortical bone.
- As age increases, an imbalance in remodelling can occur with a relative increase in bone resorption compared to bone formation.

- This results in an overall net bone loss with increased cortical porosity and loss of trabecular architecture.
- This process is particularly apparent when there is increased bone turnover, e.g. after the menopause.
- Reduced oestrogen levels cause accelerated loss of trabecular-rich bone leading to increased frequency of fractures of the vertebral bodies and distal radius over the age of 50 years.
- This is in contrast to osteomalacia which is due to defective mineralization of bone.
- More gradual age-related bone loss is associated with loss of cortical thickness. Therefore, hip fractures tend to occur later in life.

MICRO-facts

Osteoporotic fractures are more common at sites which are composed of over 50% trabecular bone and therefore most commonly affect:
- Vertebrae
- Distal radius
- Hip

MICRO-facts

- Osteoblasts make new bone. This is known as 'bone formation'.
- Osteoclasts remove bone. This is known as 'bone resorption'.
- In premenopausal disease-free states, bone formation and resorption are 'coupled', meaning that there is a steady balanced turnover of bone.

DIAGNOSIS

- Diagnosis is made using a dual energy x-ray absorptiometry (DXA) scan of the lumbar spine, hip and forearm.
- Diagnosis is based upon the World Health Organization (WHO) bone mineral density (BMD) thresholds.
- These thresholds compare an individual's BMD to the mean BMD of a young adult with the patient's bone mass being expressed as a standard deviation from the calculated peak bone mass (T-score).
- Cut-offs for the diagnostic criteria are shown in Table 17.1.

CLASSIFICATION OF OSTEOPOROSIS

- Osteoporosis can be classified as either primary or secondary.
- Primary osteoporosis includes both post-menopausal osteoporosis and involutional or age-related osteoporosis (Fig. 17.1).

Table 17.1 WHO diagnostic criteria for osteoporosis.

GROUP	WHO DIAGNOSTIC CRITERIA
Normal bone mineral density	T score, >–1 SD from the mean
Osteopaenia	BMD between –1 and –2.5 SD below the mean
Osteoporosis	BMD <–2.5 SD below the mean
Severe osteoporosis	BMD <–2.5 SD below the mean with at least 1 fragility fracture

BMD, bone mineral density; WHO, World Health Organization.

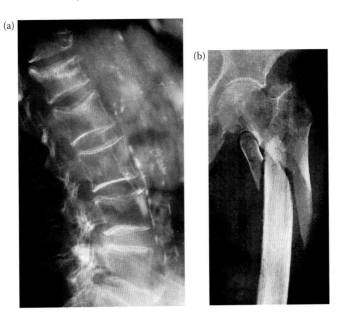

Fig. 17.1 Typical features of post-menopausal osteoporosis (a) and fracture of proximal neck of femur (b). Reproduced with permission from Solomon L, Warwick D, Nayagam S (eds.). *Apley's System of Orthopaedics and Fractures*, 9th edn. London: Hodder Arnold, 2010.

- There are several diseases, drugs and interventions which may lead to secondary osteoporosis, some of which are listed in Table 17.2.

INVESTIGATIONS

Based upon the above list, patients with osteoporosis should undergo the following investigations to rule out secondary causes and to differentiate from osteomalacia:
- Full blood count (FBC): anaemia (due to malabsorption)
- Erythrocyte sedimentation rate (ESR): multiple myeloma, rheumatoid arthritis

Table 17.2 Causes of secondary osteoporosis.

Endocrine Disorders	Malignant Disease
Hypogonadism	Multiple myeloma
Thyrotoxicosis	Leukaemia
Primary hyperparathyroidism	Lymphoma
Cushing syndrome	**Gastrointestinal**
Diabetes mellitus	Malabsorption, e.g. short bowel syndrome, coeliac disease, partial gastrectomy
Hyperprolactinaemia	**Liver disease**
Drugs	**Chronic renal disease**
Glucocorticoids	**Rheumatological**
Alcohol	Rheumatoid arthritis
Smoking	Ankylosing spondylosis
Aromatase inhibitors	**Connective tissue disorders:**
Anticonvulsants	Marfan syndrome
Androgen deprivation therapy	Ehler–Danlos syndrome
Heparin	Osteogenesis imperfecta

- Serum protein electrophoresis: multiple myeloma
- Urinary Bence–Jones proteins: multiple myeloma
- Liver function tests (LFTs): liver disease
- Serum calcium, albumin, creatinine, phosphate, alkaline phosphatase: liver disease, parathyroid disease, Paget's disease, multiple myeloma
- Thyroid function tests: thyrotoxicosis
- Anti-endomysial antibodies and anti-tissue transglutaminase antibodies: coeliac disease
- Serum prolactin: hyperprolactinaemia
- Serum testosterone, follicle-stimulating hormone (FSH), luteinizing hormone (LH), sex hormone-binding globulin (in men): androgen deficiency
- Twenty-four hour urinary cortisol/dexamethasone suppression test: Cushing syndrome
- DXA and lateral lumbar and thoracic spine radiographs
- Magnetic resonance image (MRI)/skeletal survey radiographs: multiple myeloma.

POST-MENOPAUSAL OSTEOPOROSIS

- The average age for a woman to go through the menopause is between the ages of 48 and 50 years.

- Post-menopausal osteoporosis can be attributed to the loss of oestrogen, but the cause of bone loss is multifactorial (Table 17.3).
- Oestrogen is important for controlling bone remodelling and therefore is vital for maintaining bone mass.
- Oestrogen encourages the proliferation and development of osteoblasts and decreases osteoclast formation and activity.
- Oestrogen controls osteoclast lifespan by regulating osteoclast apoptosis.
- Therefore, a decrease in oestrogen accelerates bone turnover with an imbalance in the remodelling cycle leading to a net loss of bone.
- This is known as 'uncoupling' of bone formation and resorption.
- Chronic illnesses, poor dietary intake of calcium and/or vitamin D and reduced mobility all increase the effects caused by reduced oestrogen.

TREATMENT

- The main treatment aim is to reduce the number of fractures that a patient will suffer.
- Treat any underlying cause, e.g. parathyroidectomy, in patients with primary hyperparathyroidism.
- Anti-resorptive agents are most commonly used. Once weekly bisphosphonates are the mainstay, e.g. risedronate or alendronate, although other preparations, including once monthly, once three-monthly and now even annual regimes are available.
- Catabolic or 'bone-forming' drugs are expensive and reserved for patients who continue to fracture despite treatment. Examples include teriparatide and parathyroid hormone.
- Response to treatment can be measured at 18 months using a follow-up DXA scan of the lumbar spine or by measuring markers of bone resorption or formation after four months of treatment.

Table 17.3 Risk factors for postmenopausal osteoporosis.

Caucasian or Asian ethnicity	Early onset of menopause (surgical or non-surgical)
Family history of osteoporosis. Asking about maternal hip fracture is very important	Small body habitus
History of anorexia nervosa ± amenorrhoea	Poor nutritional intake
Low peak bone mass in third decade	Lack of exercise or mobility
Alcohol intake of ≥3 units per day	Cigarette smoking

Rheumatology

MICRO-reference

National Osteoporosis Society. Glucocorticoid-induced osteoporosis. A concise guide to prevention and treatment. Available from: www.nos.org.uk/NetCommunity/Document.Doc?id=423

MICRO-print

Due to the bisphosphonate's high affinity to calcium, there is a strict set of instructions to follow in order to maximize the efficacy of the drug. These include:

- Take the tablet first thing in the morning on an empty stomach.
- Take the tablet with a full glass of tap water.
- Wait at least half an hour before having any food.
- Wait at least 1 hour before taking any other medications.
- Remain standing or at least sitting upright for at least half an hour after taking the tablet.

MICRO-case

A 65-year-old woman presents to the Emergency Department following a trip over a curb. She has sustained a Colles' fracture of her left wrist. Having treated the fracture you suspect that this patient may have osteoporosis and you refer her for an outpatient DXA bone scan.

Her bone scan reveals a T-score of −3.7 in the lumbar spine and a T-score of −3.2 at the hip. This is diagnostic of osteoporosis. As part of your investigations, you rule out any secondary causes and start a bisphosphonate with calcium and vitamin D supplement.

Points to consider

- It is important to ensure patients are vitamin D replete before commencing bisphosphonate therapy.
- A T-score of ≤2.5 SD is diagnostic of osteoporosis.
- In women over the age of 50 years, the lifetime risk of sustaining a vertebral fracture is 1 in 3 and the risk of sustaining a hip fracture is 1 in 5.

MICRO-facts

Risk factors for future fracture

- Low bone density
- Increasing age
- Female sex

continued...

continued...

- Low body mass index (BMI)
- Previous fracture, particularly of the hip, wrist or spine
- Current glucocorticoid treatment
- Current smoker
- Alcohol intake of >3 units per day

17.2 RICKETS

DEFINITION

Rickets is defined as an impaired metabolism or deficiency of vitamin D, magnesium, phosphorus or calcium and may result in a softening of bones in children. It may predispose to fractures and deformity of limbs.

EPIDEMIOLOGY

- The condition usually manifests in the first 18 months of life, although it can present for the first time during adolescence.
- Vitamin D deficiency is more common where sunlight exposure to the skin or the amount of vitamin D absorbed is reduced. For example, the malnourished, the elderly and people with dark skin.

AETIOLOGY/PATHOLOGY

- A deficiency of calcium, vitamin D or hypophosphataemia may all cause rickets.
- Failure of vitamin D metabolism may lead to rickets.
- Causes include inadequate dietary intake, lack of sunlight exposure and renal disease.
- Since there is a deficiency of the components needed to mineralize osteoid, there is a build up of unmineralized osteoid. The resulting bones are relatively weak and are unable to resist stress forces leading to deformity.

CLINICAL FEATURES

- Presentation can either be due to the disease itself or due to the symptoms and signs of complications, such as hypocalcaemia.
- Clinical features due to bone disease:
  - Skull deformity
  - Valgus deformity (knock knees)
  - Varus deformity (bowed legs) (Fig. 17.2)

Rheumatology

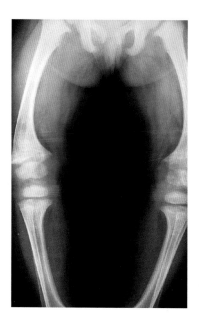

Fig. 17.2 Lower limb x-ray showing bowing of the legs. Reproduced with permission from Solomon L, Warwick D, Nayagam S (eds.). *Apley's System of Orthopaedics and Fractures*, 9th edn. London: Hodder Arnold, 2010.

- Enlargement of the costochondral junctions and physes (e.g. at the knees)
- In very severe cases, the disease may lead to fractures.
- Clinical features due to complications, such as hypocalcaemia:
  - Bone pain
  - Poor growth
  - Muscular weakness.

INVESTIGATIONS

- X-rays may show thickened and widened growth plates, bone deformity, metaphyseal cupping, 'thin' bones and erosions if secondary hyperparathyroidism is present.
- Alkaline phosphatase and parathyroid hormone may be raised, while vitamin D will be low. Calcium and phosphate may be either low or normal.
- Bone biopsy may show an excess of unmineralized osteoid though this is only performed if the diagnosis is not clear.

MANAGEMENT

Vitamin D supplements are the mainstay of treatment, although the initial cause should also be investigated and treated.

Rheumatology

17.3 OSTEOMALACIA

DEFINITION

This is effectively the same disease as rickets but occurs in adults. Therefore many of the features are similar to those of rickets; only features specific to osteomalacia will be described below.

CLINICAL FEATURES

- Patients with osteomalacia tend to have a longer history of bone pain and muscle weakness than children with rickets.
- Fractures are common.
- In contrast with rickets, there are no growth-related x-ray changes and no bowing of bones seen in osteomalacia.

INVESTIGATIONS

- X-rays: classically 'Looser's zones' can be seen which are partial fractures that have failed to heal properly.
- Isotope bone scanning reveals increased uptake at epiphyseal sites throughout the skeleton.

17.4 PAGET'S DISEASE

DEFINITION

Paget's disease is a chronic condition affecting bone remodelling. Affected bones thicken but due to the formation of disorganized bone, the overall structure is brittle.

EPIDEMIOLOGY

- Men > women (3:2).
- It is a common condition with a prevalence of 1–2% in the United States (2000).
- The disease is uncommon under 40 years.
- Prevalence increases with increasing age.
- Prevalence varies in different counties. While it is common in countries such as Britain and Australia, it is uncommon in Africa.

> **MICRO-reference**
> Altman R D, Bloch D A, Hochberg M C, Murphy W A. Prevalence of pelvic Paget's disease of bone in the United States. *Journal of Bone and Mineral Research* 2000; 15: 461–5.

AETIOLOGY

The aetiology of Paget's disease is unknown; both genetic and infectious components are postulated.

- Genetics:
  - Genes and mutations have been postulated in the aetiology of Paget's disease.
  - First-degree relatives of a person with Paget's disease have a seven-fold increased chance of developing the disease.
- Infection:
  - In reality, it is probably a combination of these hypotheses which causes the disease to manifest.

PATHOGENESIS

- The key element of the pathogenesis of Paget's disease is abnormal bone remodeling.
- Primarily, large osteoclasts are activated and resorb bone at a higher rate than in normal subjects.
- Osteoblasts then produce new woven and lamellar bone in a disorganized fashion so it is structurally weak.
- This process of bone resorption and formation continues so that the resulting bone is thicker than it was previously, but also more brittle.
- In the later stages of the disease, the bone is sclerotic.

CLINICAL FEATURES

- There may be none.
- Bone pain of an achy nature; more severe if a fracture is present.
- Skeletal deformities (bowing of lower limb bones, kyphosis in patients with spinal involvement).
- Skin is warmer over the affected bones than on other parts of the body.
- In cases where the skull is involved: the calvarium is thickened so the head changes shape and gets bigger. The base of the skull also flattens.
- Nerve compression resulting from Paget's disease in the vertebrae or skull which causes complications such as cranial nerve palsies.

PATHOLOGICAL FRACTURES

- Steal syndrome: blood is 'stolen' from organs and taken to the skeletal circulation instead. This can lead to complications, such as cerebral impairment.
- Formation of osteosarcoma in Pagetic bone is a well-recognized, if uncommon, complication. The affected bone will appear painful, swollen and tender.

MICRO-facts

Pagetic fractures pose increased risk of serious haemorrhage due to their increased vascularity.

MICRO-facts

Sites usually affected by Paget's disease: skull, clavicle, vertebrae, pelvis, femur, tibia.

MICRO-facts

In patients with Paget's disease affecting the skull, cranial nerves can become compressed and the following complications may arise: deafness, visual impairment, trigeminal neuralgia and facial palsy.

MICRO-case

Mrs Pagète is a 75-year-old woman who presents to her GP. She is feeling rather anxious because none of her hats will fit on her head anymore and her friends have commented that her face seems to have changed shape. She also says that her hearing has deteriorated over the past few months and she wants to know what is causing all these problems. After investigation, the GP diagnoses the patient with Paget's disease.

Points to consider

- The patient describes signs of Paget's disease involving the skull.
- Her head has increased in size and shape due to thickening of the bone.
- Her hearing could be reduced for one of two complications that occur in Paget's disease:
  - Compression of the auditory nerve by newly formed bone
  - Otosclerosis.

MICRO-print

Calcium levels are usually normal in Paget's. However, there is a predisposition to develop secondary hyperparathyroidism, which is thought to be due to dietary intake of calcium not meeting the increased demand by Pagetic bone.

Rheumatology

INVESTIGATIONS

- Blood tests:
  - Serum alkaline phosphatase ↑
  - Serum calcium
- Imaging:
  - Plain x-rays
  - Isotope bone scan (Table 17.4).
- Serum alkaline phosphatase is a very useful test in Paget's disease as it reveals the level of activity of the disease: the higher the alkaline phosphatase, the more active the disease.
- Note: bone alkaline phosphatase is different from liver alkaline phosphatase so a raised alkaline phosphatase is only diagnostic of Paget's in the appropriate clinical context.

COMPLICATIONS

- Nerve compression and osteosarcoma are complications that have been discussed previously in this chapter (see above under Pathological fractures) because they may be presenting features of Paget's disease in some patients.
- Fractures can be complete and occur in the long bones, or they can be microfractures on the convex surface of a bowed bone. Both of these types of fracture can produce pain and microfractures can worsen to become complete fractures.
- Hypercalcaemia.
- Osteoarthritis can occur in joints that involve a bone affected by Paget's disease.
- High output cardiac failure is caused by the increased blood flow in the Pagetic bone.

Table 17.4 **Results in patients with Paget's disease.**

INVESTIGATION	RESULT IN PATIENTS WITH PAGET'S DISEASE
Alkaline phosphatase	↑
X-rays	Variable depending on stage of disease:
	Patches of osteoporosis
	Osteolytic areas: a flame shaped lesion in bones
	Areas of sclerosis
	Thickened bone
	Coarse trabeculation
	Fractures
Isotope bone scan	↑ Uptake in bones affected by disease

MANAGEMENT

- For some patients with localized disease, no treatment is necessary.
- Regular appointments: serum alkaline phosphatase should be measured regularly. Changes in symptoms should prompt reassessment of the patient including examination, appropriate investigations and a medication review.
- Medications: bisphosphonates or calcitonin. Both these drugs work by altering the rate of bone turnover and can markedly improve symptoms.
- Surgical options: these are only considered when complications develop, such as pathological fractures which usually need fixing surgically.
    - Neurological complications, such as nerve compression and spinal stenosis, will need treating by decompression surgery.
    - If an osteosarcoma develops in Pagetic bone, it may be possible to amputate the limb where the tumour is present but prognosis remains poor.
    - Osteotomy is sometimes performed to correct bone deformities, such as bowing.

MICRO-case

Mr Clast is a 50-year-old man who presents with pain in his left leg which then becomes localized to the shin. On examination, the doctor notes that the skin over the patient's leg feels a great deal warmer than the skin over other areas of his body. Paget's disease is high on the doctor's list of differential diagnoses. Investigations are performed which confirm the diagnosis.

Points to consider

- Alkaline phosphatase would be raised and is also helpful in that it gives an indication of the level of activity of the disease.
- X-rays may show different changes depending on the stage of disease, but common abnormalities include areas of sclerosis, thickened bone and fractures, among other signs.
- An isotope bone scan would show an increased area of uptake in Pagetic bones.

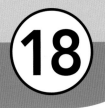

Bone and joint infection

18.1 SEPTIC ARTHRITIS

DEFINITION

Septic arthritis is defined as bacterial infection within the joint space.

AETIOLOGY AND PATHOPHYSIOLOGY

The causative organism is usually *Staphylococcus aureus*.

CLINICAL FEATURES

Septic arthritis presents as a warm, painful, swollen joint.

INVESTIGATIONS

- White cell count (WCC) and C-reactive protein (CRP) are elevated.
- Aspiration of the joint may reveal pus in the joint space. This should be sent for microscopy, culture and sensitivity.
- If the patient has a prosthetic joint, then it is vital that an orthopaedic surgeon is contacted as the aspiration will need to take place in theatre to minimize risk of introducing infection.

MANAGEMENT

- Systemic antibiotics should be started urgently and the joint washed out in theatre.
- Empirical antibiotics, such as flucloxacillin, are used until sensitivities are known.

18.2 OSTEOMYELITIS

DEFINITION

Osteomyelitis is defined as an infection of the bone marrow or bone itself.

EPIDEMIOLOGY

The epidemiology is unknown.

AETIOLOGY/PATHOPHYSIOLOGY

- The causes of osteomyelitis depend on age group, but the common causative organisms in all age groups are *Staphylococcus aureus*, *Streptococcus* spp. and *Enterococcus* spp.
- The route of infectious transmission can be direct by exposure of a specific bone either through trauma or perioperatively (hence the extra precautions, such as full hoods that surgeons take during orthopaedic operations).
- Other at risk patients include intravenous drug users, the immunosuppressed and dental patients where causative organisms can spread by a haematogenous route.

CLINICAL FEATURES

- Bone: pain, erythema, swelling, warm to touch, loss of movement.
- Overlying trauma or scabbing.
- Systemic features, such as fever, malaise and lethargy.

INVESTIGATIONS

- X-ray shows a lytic core with surrounding sclerosis.
- Blood and joint aspirate cultures should be taken for microscopy, cytology and sensitivities.

MANAGEMENT

- Long-term course of antibiotics (typically a 6–8-week course). The intravenous route is normally the route of choice.
- Debridement of the affected area.

18.3 TUBERCULOSIS

DEFINITION

- Tuberculosis (TB) is an infectious mycobacterium disease which is passed by droplet spread from person to person. The majority of sufferers are asymptomatic (and latent).
- This section concentrates on infection of the bone with *Mycobacterium tuberculosis*.

EPIDEMIOLOGY

- TB used to be a main cause of death in the UK, but the prevalence gradually declined due to better living conditions, pasteurization of milk and management of the disease with an all-time low level of cases in the 1980s.
- Since then, the prevalence has increased slightly in certain UK communities, but the disease is still not common in the UK.

AETIOLOGY/PATHOPHYSIOLOGY

- TB is caught by inhalation of particles produced when someone with the active infection coughs or sneezes. The disease then spreads into other organs, such as bone.
- Prolonged exposure is usually necessary for infection to develop.
- The risk of catching the disease is increased in certain people, for example, those who are malnourished, immunocompromised or who have lived in a country where the disease is prevalent.
- The disease can reactivate from the primary lesion.

CLINICAL FEATURES

- Patients may have the classical generalized symptoms of TB, such as weight loss, haemoptysis, night sweats and cough.
- If the infection has spread to the bone, they will give a history of a gradual onset of pain.

EXAMINATION (WITH RELATION TO TB OF THE BONE)

- The whole joint may be destroyed causing pain in and around the area, often including the iliac fossa.
- Commonly an abscess will be present and spinal movements will also be restricted.

INVESTIGATIONS

- To diagnose TB infection in bone, samples of the affected areas need to be taken and cultured.
- If the infection is present, a Ziehl–Neelsen stain of a sample will show red alcohol-fast mycobacterium.
- X-rays will show periarticular osteopenia and destruction of the bone.

MANAGEMENT

- This will include anti-TB medication and rest/support in plaster.
- Later treatment when pain has been managed may include arthrodesis.

19 Bone tumours

Tumours specific to different bones are covered in the relevant chapters. Here we cover multiple myeloma and bone metastases.

19.1 MULTIPLE MYELOMA

DEFINITION

Multiple myeloma is a malignancy of plasma cells.

EPIDEMIOLOGY

The disease usually presents in people over the age of 60 years, but may occur in much younger adults.

AETIOLOGY

- The disease progresses from an expansion of malignant plasma cells in the bone marrow.
- Common sites affected by the disease are the vertebrae, ribs and clavicles.

CLINICAL FEATURES

- Patients with multiple myeloma may have features of bone marrow failure such as anaemia, neutropenia or thrombocytopenia.
- Corresponding symptoms such as fatigue, increased susceptibility to infection and spontaneous bleeding may be present.
- Due to the bone involvement, patients often present with bone pain, pathological fractures, nerve compression syndromes or symptoms of hypercalcaemia.
- Myeloma may also be complicated by renal failure.

INVESTIGATIONS

- X-rays of affected bones may show lytic areas (typically described as 'punched out') (Fig. 19.1). The erythrocyte sedimentation rate (ESR) is usually elevated; urea, creatinine and calcium may also be raised.
- Electrophoresis of the serum reveals a paraprotein band. Urine electropheresis reveals Bence-Jones protein or 'light chains', and bone marrow biopsy shows a plasma cell infiltrate.

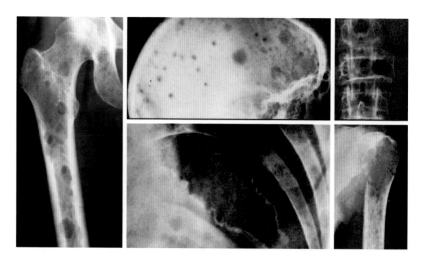

Fig. 19.1 X-ray features of multiple myeloma. Reproduced with permission from Solomon L, Warwick D, Nayagam S. *Apley's System of Orthopaedics and Fractures*, 9th edn. London: Hodder Arnold, 2010.

MANAGEMENT

- Chemotherapy is the main method of treatment. In fit patients, autologous or allogenic stem cell transplantation may be considered.
- Bone involvement is treated with bisphosphonates.
- Treat complications of the disease, such as anaemia and renal failure, with appropriate management.

PROGNOSIS

Myeloma has a very poor prognosis with survival averaging between three and four years.

19.2 BONE METASTASES

DEFINITION

Bone metastases are defined as spread of malignancy from a primary site to bone.

> **MICRO-print**
> Symptoms from bone metastases may be the first presentation of a malignancy, so it is important that the patient is appropriately investigated for a primary source.

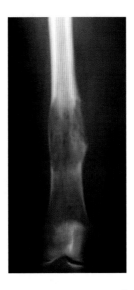

Fig. 19.2 Metastatic femoral bone lesion. Reproduced with permission from Williams N, Bulstrode C, O'Connell R. *Bailey & Love's Short Practice of Surgery*, 26th edn. London: Hodder Arnold, 2013.

AETIOLOGY

- There are a number of known cancers that commonly metastasize to bone. Often they will localize to the vertebrae, ribs, humerus, pelvis or femur.
- Spread may be haematogenous or by direct spread.
- The metastases initiate bone destruction either by direct action, or by altering the fine balance between osteoclastic bone resorption and osteoblastic bone formation.
- Metastases are usually osteolytic in nature, apart from prostate metastases which are sclerotic.

MICRO-facts

Cancers that commonly metastasize to bone are:
- Breast
- Prostate
- Thyroid
- Lung
- Kidney

CLINICAL FEATURES

- Symptoms of the primary malignancy may be present, such as haemoptysis in lung cancer.

- Bone pain is a common presentation. Other clinical features include bone fractures from low impact forces, symptoms of hypercalcaemia and nerve compression (Fig. 19.2).

INVESTIGATIONS

- X-rays may highlight lesions in the bone or bone destruction and fractures.
- White cell count (WCC), C-reactive protein (CRP), erythrocyte sedimentation rate (ESR), alkaline phosphatase, calcium and specific cancer markers, such as prostate specific antigen (PSA) may be raised.
- Haemoglobin may be low.
- Isotope bone scan may show the locations of bony metastases as 'hot spots'.
- Magnetic resonance image (MRI) may be used to monitor the disease and to identify further metastases.
- If the primary malignancy is unknown, appropriate investigations should be performed to identify this.

MANAGEMENT

- Pain needs to be managed carefully, using opioids if necessary. It may be appropriate to refer the patient to the pain clinic.
- Radiotherapy can reduce bone pain and halt tumour growth.
- Treatment of the primary may be possible. For example, in patients with primary breast cancer, the tumour may be responsive to hormone therapy.
- Fracture treatment should be performed and impending fractures should also be stabilized.
- Bisphosphonates are also prescribed to patients with bony metastases to reduce hypercalcaemia.

MICRO-case

Ms Rose is a 53-year-old woman who is usually fit and well. However, over the last two months she has been having some tenderness around her rib cage. Initially, she was thought to have pleurisy, but after further investigations the diagnosis was changed to costochondritis. A month later when her symptoms had still not improved, her GP noticed she had lost some weight and she complained of being tired all the time. A serum calcium level was taken which was found to be elevated. The patient was found to have bone metastases from an unknown primary.

Points to consider
- Since the primary is unknown, appropriate investigations will need to be undertaken to diagnose the malignancy.
- This woman will also need blood taken for a full blood count (FBC), CRP, ESR and alkaline phosphatase levels, a bone scan to identify areas of bone affected by metastases, and x-rays of the affected bones. An MRI may also be indicated.

Rheumatology

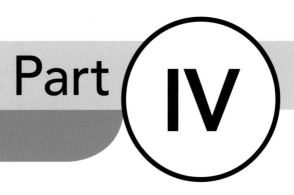

Part IV

Self-assessment

20 Orthopaedics

HEAD AND NECK QUESTIONS

In each of the following clinical situations, you must choose the most likely diagnosis. Each option may be used once, more than once or not at all.

DIAGNOSTIC OPTIONS

1. C2 fracture
2. C5 fracture
3. Disc prolapse
4. Erb's palsy
5. Le Fort type I
6. Le Fort type II
7. Osteoarthritis
8. Posterior fossa trauma
9. Rheumatoid arthritis
10. Tibial plate fracture

Question 1

You are the Emergency Department junior doctor on call at night. You have been fast-bleeped to go to the resuscitation unit to see a 35-year-old man who has fallen downstairs in a pub and been brought in by the paramedics. The patient has a Guedel (oropharyngeal airway) in situ and a Glasgow Coma Score (GCS) of 8. While he is being stabilized by your registrar and the nursing staff, you notice what looks like bruising behind an ear. What might the bruising a sign of?

Question 2

While working as a junior doctor in the Emergency Department, a 21-year-old male who has been in a road traffic accident (RTA) presents with a GCS of 3. The anaesthetist attempts to bag and mask the patient, but realizes the chest is not rising and reassesses the airway immediately. When you inspect the head and neck, you realize that the mechanism of injury is frontal facial trauma. You suggest an emergency mini-tracheostomy. The anaesthetist agrees and completes the procedure. Why?

Question 3

You have some free time from work and decide to watch a local rugby match. During the game, the scrum collapses. All but one of the players stands up again to reset the scrum. You run onto the pitch and tell the players not to move the player. You immediately stabilize his neck and assess the player's ABC (airway, breathing, circulation) (which are present). He has a GCS of 15. What were you worried about?

Question 4

You are sitting your medical school finals and the examiner asks you to examine the patient's upper limb. While examining the patient, you note he has a scar on his neck and a left C5/6 palsy. Which sign(s) might have led you to this diagnosis?

1. Biceps hyperreflexia
2. Resisted passive wrist extension
3. 'Shoulder badge' anaesthesia
4. Small muscle wasting in the hand
5. The 'waiter's tip' sign

Question 5

Which of the following is a sign of brachial plexus injury following neck trauma?

1. Compartment syndrome
2. Corrigan's sign
3. Erb's palsy
4. Bulbar palsy
5. Klumpke's paralysis

THORACIC AND LUMBAR SPINE QUESTIONS

For each of the following clinical scenarios, all of which focus on the thoracolumbar spine, please choose the most likely diagnosis. Each option may be used once, more than once or not at all.

Question 1

You are called to see a patient who has recently undergone a knee arthroscopy under a spinal anaesthetic. His knee is much better, but he is pyrexial and very tender on his back at the level of L3/L4. You suspect discitis. What organism are his blood cultures likely to grow?

1. *Haemophylus influenzae*
2. *Mycobacterium tuberculosus*
3. *Pseudomonas aeruginosa*
4. *Staphyloccus aureus*
5. *Streptococcus pneumoniae*

Question 2

A 40-year-old man is brought to the Emergency Department at 4 p.m. by his wife. He feels fine except his wife has noticed he has been stumbling around today. The man admits that he also has a strange tingling sensation down the back of both legs and they feel numb. On general examination, you notice an area of dullness to percussion above the symphysis pubis. What investigation do you order?

1. Abdominal x-ray
2. Chest x-ray
3. MRI (magnetic resonance image)
4. PET-CT (positron emission tomography-computed tomography)
5. USS (ultrasound) pelvis

Question 3

You are working in the city centre as a trainee GP and your next patient is a 36-year-old man originally from Nigeria. He was diagnosed with HIV six months ago while still in Nigeria and is not currently taking any medication. He complains of feeling lethargic and generally unwell for the past few months. He also complains of having back pain, which came on at a similar time to his other symptoms. What is the likely cause of his back pain and other symptoms?

1. Cauda equina syndrome
2. Vertebral fracture
3. Spinal stenosis
4. Spinal tuberculosis
5. Spinal tumour.

Question 4

Which is the most common level at which spondylolisthesis occurs?

1. C6/C7
2. L3/L4
3. L5/S1
4. S1/S2
5. T10/T11

Question 5

A 12-year-old girl presents in clinic with a spinal deformity. There is an obvious lateral curvature to the spine. You make a diagnosis of adolescent idiopathic scoliosis and want to measure the Cobb angle. What imaging method is best for this?

1. AP (anteroposterior) x-ray
2. CT (computed tomography)
3. MRI
4. PA (posteroanterior) x-ray
5. USS

SHOULDER QUESTIONS

For each of the following clinical scenarios, all of which focus on the shoulder, please choose the most likely diagnosis. Each option may be used once, more than once or not at all.

DIAGNOSTIC OPTIONS:

1. Anterior shoulder dislocation
2. Deep vein thrombosis (DVT)
3. Fracture of proximal humeral head
4. Impingement syndrome
5. Osteosarcoma
6. Pneumonia
7. Posterior shoulder dislocation
8. Pulmonary embolus
9. Supraspinatus injury
10. Teres minor injury

Question 1

You are a junior doctor on call at night and have been phoned by a ward sister to see a 79-year-old man who is 5 days post-op from an elective shoulder replacement. He is short of breath, which has been progressively worse over the last 3 hours, with a non-productive cough.

Of note from his background history you identify that he is a retired plasterer and has well-controlled asthma with a BMI (body mass index) of 34.

On examination you find him apyrexial, tachypnoeic and tachycardic with vescicular breath sounds.

Question 2

You are on an orthopaedic ward round and you are asked by the consultant to examine the rotator cuff of a female patient. You test all the rotator cuff muscles and elicit a positive sign when the patient attempts to perform abduction with elbow by their side against resistance.

Question 3

Whilst on a shift in the Emergency Department, a 28-year-old male judo expert presents holding his arm across his torso and complaining of sudden severe shoulder pain. On examination, there is a loss of sensation over the C5 dermatome.

Question 4

You are on an orthopaedic revision course and the teacher asks you to examine a patient at the front of the lecture theatre. While actively moving the patient's arm in abduction, you find they have pain suggestive of impingement syndrome. This pain is likely to be:

1. 60–120°
2. 0–90°

3. Full arc
4. Pain on palpation of the acromioclavicular (AC) joint
5. 120–180°.

Question 5

Which of the following is not a muscle forming the rotator cuff?
1. Supraspinatus
2. Teres major
3. Subscapularis
4. Infraspinatus
5. Teres minor

ELBOW QUESTIONS

For each of the following clinical scenarios, all of which focus on the elbow, please choose the most likely diagnosis. Each option may be used once, more than once or not at all.

DIAGNOSTIC OPTIONS:

1. Golfer's elbow
2. Gout
3. Loose body
4. Median nerve palsy
5. Osteoarthritis

6. Posterior ulno-humeral dislocation
7. Rheumatoid arthritis
8. Supra-condylar fracture
9. Tennis elbow
10. Ulnar nerve palsy

Question 1

You are a junior doctor in general practice. The first patient of the morning is a 43-year-old right-handed man who has promised his wife he will lose some weight. He has been working very hard at this, taking up several sports over the last six months including golf and tennis. However, he has had to slow down over the last couple of weeks as he is complaining of a painful elbow which on examination appears to be particularly tender over the lateral epicondyle. He is otherwise well.

Question 2

You are on an orthopaedic ward round and you are asked to examine the neurological status of the upper limb in a 34-year-old man who suffered a severe intra-articular fracture of his right elbow. He is now 2 days post-operation. You find that he is unable to abduct, nor oppose his thumb. He has reduced sensation in his thumb, index finger, middle finger and radial aspect of his ring finger.

Question 3

While on a shift in the Emergency Department, a 7-year-old boy is brought in by his parents having fallen over onto an outstretched hand. He is in a great deal of pain making examination difficult. However, you are able to feel that the bony landmarks are abnormal, but that the elbow joint is not dislocated.

Question 4

You are asked by your consultant to present an x-ray of a patient with osteoarthritis of the elbow. Which of the following features will not be present?
1. Bone cysts
2. Destruction of soft tissues
3. Joint space narrowing
4. Osteophytes
5. Subarticular sclerosis.

Question 5

Which of the following is not commonly fractured with a dislocation of the elbow?
1. Coracoid process
2. Coronoid process
3. Medial epicondyle
4. Olecranon process
5. Radial head.

HAND AND WRIST QUESTIONS

For each of the following clinical scenarios, all of which focus on the hand and wrist, choose the most likely diagnosis. Each option may be used once, more than once, or not at all.

DIAGNOSTIC OPTIONS:

1. Barton's fracture
2. Colles' fracture
3. De Quervain's disease
4. Dupuytren's disease
5. Ganglion

6. Mallet finger
7. Paget's disease
8. Scaphoid fracture
9. Tenosynovitis
10. Trigger finger

Question 1

You are the junior doctor working on call in orthopaedics at the weekend. You get called down to the Emergency Department to see a 26-year-old right-handed male who has injured his finger during a cricket match. On examination, the only deformity is that the terminal phalanx of the patient's right index finger is dropped compared to the others and he cannot straighten it. What is the injury he is likely to have sustained?

Question 2

A 45-year-old woman presents to the Emergency Department following a fall onto her hand. After examining her, you have a working diagnosis and take appropriate x-rays but you cannot see a fracture on the films. However, you are keen to follow this woman up closely because you are aware of the complications that could occur if the patient did indeed have the condition you suspect. What is the most likely pathology?

Question 3

Mr Fascia is a 50-year-old man who presents to the orthopaedic hand clinic. He has been referred by his general practitioner because he has noticed that his right ring finger will not straighten out as much as it used to and it is causing him some functional disability. He recalls that his father had the same symptoms. What is the likely diagnosis?

Question 4

A 50-year-old right-handed woman presents to the orthopaedic hand clinic complaining of pins and needles in her right hand in the middle of the night. You think the diagnosis may be carpal tunnel syndrome, but want to perform the most sensitive test for the disease on the patient. Which of the following do you choose to do?

1. Durkin's test
2. Finkelstein's test
3. Ortolani test
4. Phalen's test
5. Tinel's test

Question 5

Mr Gunn is a 44-year-old man who presents to the orthopaedic hand clinic because he has been having problems moving his left ring finger. He says that when he straightens it, it catches and then suddenly extends. His only past medical history of note is diabetes mellitus. What is the likely diagnosis of this patient's finger problem?

1. Dupuytren's disease
2. Mallet finger
3. Osteoarthritis
4. Radial nerve lesion
5. Trigger finger

SACRUM AND PELVIS QUESTIONS

For each of the following clinical scenarios, all of which focus on the sacrum and pelvis, please choose the most likely diagnosis. Each option may be used once, more than once or not at all.

DIAGNOSTIC OPTIONS:

1. Acetabular fracture	6. Osteomalacia
2. Ankylosing spondylitis	7. Pelvic ring fracture
3. Avulsion fracture	8. Sacral fracture
4. Chondrosarcoma	9. Tuberculosis
5. Osteochondroma	10. Urethral injury

Question 1

You are the junior doctor in general practice. A 20-year-old man comes to see you because he has been having some pain and stiffness in his hip and pelvis, usually worse in the morning. On examination, you note that he is tender over this area. What is an important differential?

Question 2

A 45-year-man who has recently moved from Bangladesh to England presents to the Emergency Department. You are the junior doctor working there and you see this man. After taking a history, you find out that he has had a productive cough for about 6 weeks, lost about 12 kg in weight over the last couple of months, is experiencing night sweats, and has pain in his groin and iliac fossa on the left side. What condition do you need to test this man for?

Question 3

A 25-year-old female zookeeper in charge of the indoor bat cave has an appointment to see you, the junior doctor at a general practice. She presents with bony pelvic pain. There is no other information of note in the history apart from the fact that she is a strict vegan. Based on this information, what diagnosis would you consider in this woman?

Question 4

A 30-year-old man is brought into the Emergency Department following a head-on collision with a wall while he was a passenger in a car. The car was travelling at approximately 30 mph on impact with the wall. He has a GCS of 15/15, but is complaining of severe pain in his hip region. After imaging, you find he has an acetabular fracture. What complication is commonly associated with this type of fracture?

1. Osteoarthritis
2. Compartment syndrome
3. Avascular necrosis
4. Recurrent dislocation of the femoral head
5. Chronic bleeding from the fracture site.

Question 5

You are a doctor working in the Emergency Department. A 50-year-old male pedestrian is brought in by the ambulance crew following a collision at 60 mph with a car. After initial management you examine him and find that there is blood around the urethral meatus. You are concerned that he may have a urethral injury. What further examination could you do to investigate this suspicion?

1. Digital rectal examination (DRE)
2. Hip examination
3. Lumbar spine examination
4. Regional examination of the musculoskeletal system
5. Testicular examination.

HIP QUESTIONS

For each of the following clinical scenarios, all of which focus on the hip, please choose the most likely diagnosis. Each option may be used once, more than once or not at all.

DIAGNOSTIC OPTIONS:

1. Adam's test
2. Barlow's manoeurve
3. DXA
4. ESR blood test
5. Evan's test
6. Ortolani's test
7. Parling's manoeurve
8. Rheumatoid Arthritis
9. Thomas' test
10. Trendelenburg test

Question 1

You are a junior doctor in an orthopaediatric clinic. A mother brings her 18-month-old son to see you. She tells you that she is worried because her son has not started to crawl. You note from his background history that the family has recently arrived in the UK from Bangladesh. On examination, you find the child is apyrexial. When examining the hips, you illicit a positive response when you put forward pressure on his left groin. What test did you perform?

Question 2

You are the on-call orthopaedic junior doctor and you have been bleeped by an Accident and Emergency nurse. An 85-year-old woman has presented with a fall and chest pain. You are concerned about osteoporosis. What test or investigation could you perform to confirm your suspicion?

Question 3

You are teaching a group of third-year medical students who are on placement with your firm. They ask how would you prevent the pelvis from masking hip flexion deformity when assessing the range of movement of the hip? Which test do you show them?

Question 4

In hip pathology, which muscle is responsible for the shortening and lateral rotation of the leg?
1. Gluteus medius
2. Gluteus minimus
3. Pectineus
4. Psoas
5. Quadriceps femoris.

Question 5

You are at an orthopaedic conference workshop. You are asked to examine a volunteer for adduction of the hip. The consultant running the workshop asks you what is the normal range of movement in a healthy patient?
1. 0–30°
2. 0–50°
3. 0–60°
4. 0–140°
5. 25–140°.

KNEE QUESTIONS

For each of the following clinical scenarios, all of which focus on the knee, please choose the most likely diagnosis. Each option may be used once, more than once or not at all.

DIAGNOSTIC OPTIONS:

1. Anterior cruciate ligament
2. Dislocation of the patella
3. Medial collateral ligament
4. Meniscal tear
5. Osteoarthritis
6. Osteochondritis dissecans
7. Popliteal cyst
8. Popliteal aneurysm
9. Posterior cruciate ligament
10. Tibial plateau fracture

Question 1

You are working in general practice and your next patient is a 22-year-old man. He is fit and well and regularly plays sport, but has recently noticed that his left knee swells after football and has a dull ache afterwards. He denies any locking of the joint.

Question 2

A 68-year-old man comes to your practice complaining that he now shuffles his right foot along the floor while walking as it 'doesn't work properly'. He has also noticed a lump over the posterior aspect of his knee. On examination, you find that he has foot drop, as well as a pulsatile mass behind the right knee.

Question 3

The next case you see in the Emergency Department is of a 23-year-old rugby player who has come in supported by two of his teammates as he cannot walk. He plays on the wing and was in the process of sidestepping a player when he felt a sudden snap and immediate pain in his knee which swelled dramatically over the next few minutes. On examination, there is a diffuse swelling and the knee is very painful. Aspiration of the joint reveals a haemarthrosis.

Question 4

Which of the following is not a risk factor for recurrent patella dislocation:
1. A deep trochlear groove
2. A small patella
3. High riding patella (*patella alta*)
4. Ligamentous laxity
5. Valgus deformity of the knee.

Question 5

A Sunday league footballer is taking a direct free kick, however as he goes to take the kick he twists his knee and feels immediate pain over the medial aspect of his knee. He is unable to continue because of this, but he also finds that his knee is locked. What is the most likely affected structure?
1. Anterior cruciate ligament (ACL)
2. Lateral collateral ligament (LCL)
3. Medial collateral ligament (MCL)
4. Medial meniscus
5. Posterior cruciate ligament (PCL)

ANKLE AND FOOT QUESTIONS

Please choose the most likely answer in each of the following clinical scenarios. An option may be used once, more than once or not at all.

DIAGNOSTIC OPTIONS:

1. Dorisflex
2. Equinovalgus
3. Equinovarus
4. Evert
5. Extend
6. Invert
7. Plantarflex
8. Plantigrade
9. Planus
10. Rotate

Question 1

You are a volunteer doctor at an athletic event. A runner is brought to your station on a stretcher complaining of sudden onset of excruciating left calf pain while running in the 200 metre sprint.

As part of your clinical examination you perform Simmond's test, which is negative for an Achilles tendon rupture. What did you do and look for that confirmed a negative test result?

Question 2

During a paediatric orthopaedic clinic, an anxious mother brings her five-month-old boy to see you after being referred by the family GP. The GP states in his referral letter that when he examined the child he had bilateral club feet. You examine the boy and agree with the GP's findings. How were the child's feet positioned to be classed as club feet?

Question 3

You have just started your new rotation as an anatomy demonstrator and you are leading a dissection session on the lower limb. One of the medical students asks you how the anterior talofibular ligament of the ankle can be injured. What is your reply?

Question 4

In the Salter-Harris classification, which type of fracture is a fracture through the physis, metaphysis and epiphysis?
1. I
2. II
3. III
4. IV
5. V

Question 5

Which one of the following is not part of the Ottawa ankle and foot rules?
1. Calcaneal tenderness
2. Fifth metatarsal base (styloid) tenderness
3. Lateral malleolar tenderness
4. Medial malleolar tenderness
5. Unable to weight bear.

ANSWERS TO HEAD AND NECK QUESTIONS

Answer 1

(8) Posterior fossa. The patient has Battle's sign. This is a retromastoid bruise that is highly suggestive of a posterior fossa fracture.

Answer 2

(6) Le Fort type II. A frontal high energy mechanism of injury such as a high speed RTA can result in major trauma including a Le Fort type II maxillary fracture. The injury had compromised the pharyngeal airway by depressing the maxilla into the facial skeleton so occluding the airway. An emergency mini-tracheostomy can be life-saving in these cases.

Answer 3

(2) C5 fracture: All contact sports carry the risk of catastrophic injury. It is better to have a cautious approach to this type of rugby injury even if the player has a GCS 15 and wants to play on. You must rule out possible occult sinister pathology, which in this case might have been a C5 fracture (a not uncommon rugby scrum injury). This level of injury might also compromise ventilation (remember 'C3, 4, 5, keeps the diaphragm alive').

Answer 4

(5) The 'waiter's tip' sign: The 'waiter's tip' sign indicating upper brachial cord injury (Erb's palsy). C5/6 lower motor neurone (LMN) injury causes paralysis or variable weakness of deltoid, brachialis and biceps muscle function. LMN involvement causes biceps hyporeflexia. Shoulder internal and forearm flexor power dominates (C7, 8) causing the 'waiter's tip' sign. The extent of sensory loss can vary from the local 'regimental badge' (C5, circumflex) to more extensive and increasing upper arm and forearm antero/postero and latero/medial hypoaesthesia.

Answer 5

(5) Klumpke's paralysis. This is a brachial plexus lower cord injury (C8 and T1). Often found when a motorcyclist has been involved in a collision when their neck and shoulders are violently abducted. The arm is adducted with paralysis of the intrinsic muscles of the hand, decreased sensation in the ulnar territory and sometimes Horner's syndrome (ptosis, meiosis, enopthalmos and anhidrosis).

ANSWERS TO THORACIC AND LUMBAR SPINE QUESTIONS

Answer 1

(4) *Staphylococcus aureus*. Most discitis is due to haematogenous spread from a distant site or through the introduction of bacteria during an invasive procedure on the spine. *Staphylococcus aureus* is the most common causative organism as this is the predominant microorganism on the skin.

Answer 2

(3) MRI. This is the most appropriate imaging technique for visualizing the location and extent of the spinal pathology. MRI is the best radiological investigation for assessing soft tissue.

Answer 3

(4) Spinal tuberculosis. In an immunocompromised patient recently arrived from a tuberculosis (TB) endemic area, the clinician must be highly suspicious of TB and must exclude this diagnosis in at risk patients.

Answer 4

(3) L5/S1. Spondylolisthesis means a slipped vertebra. It involves the forward displacement of one vertebral body on the vertebra below. It most commonly occurs between the L5/S1 or L4/L5 vertebral bodies.

Answer 5

(4) PA x-ray. The angle of the curve is measured on the full length standing posteroanterior (PA) spine x-ray and is called Cobb's angle.

ANSWERS TO SHOULDER QUESTIONS

Answer 1

(8) Pulmonary embolism. Classical signs of a pulmonary embolism (PE) include dyspnoea, cough with or without haemoptysis, tachycardia, arrhythmia, sudden death, hypotension, engorged neck veins, right ventricular gallop, pleuritic chest pain, preceding leg pain, raised jugular venous pressure (JVP), cyanosis. Any post-operative patient is at an increased risk. Note that the past medical history of well controlled asthma is actually a red herring!

Answer 2

(9) Supraspinatus injury. Abduction with the elbow by the side against resistance isolates the supraspinatus muscle and elicits a painful response if the muscle is damaged.

- Rotator cuff muscle function:
- Supraspinatus – initial abduction
- Infraspinatus – external rotation
- Subscapularis – internal rotation
- Teres minor – external rotation.

Answer 3

(1) Anterior dislocation of the shoulder. Patient often presents holding injured arm in the other hand across the chest. Sudden severe pain with loss of deltoid bulk and a small bulge may be palpated below the clavicle. It is important to check sensation over the 'regimental badge' distribution before and after reduction of the joint because of the risk of damage to the axillary nerve.

Answer 4

(1) 60–120°. This range of movement causes maximum stress on the rotator cuff tendons passing through the narrow space between the head of the humerus and the acromium. Causes include trauma, calcification, spurs and inflammation.

Answer 5

(2) Teres major. This muscle is not classed as a rotator cuff muscle, however, it is one of the scapulohumeral muscles and is responsible for aiding the latissimus dorsi in the action of pulling the humerus down and back from an elevated position.

ANSWERS TO ELBOW QUESTIONS

Answer 1

(9) Tennis elbow affects the lateral epicondyle. There may also be swelling over this area and a loss of extension. It may be aggravated by lifting heavy objects and shaking hands.

Answer 2

(4) This describes a median nerve palsy. The level of damage determines the palsy seen. Injuries to the nerve occurring distally result in paralysis of the thenar muscles and the first and second lumbricals. Sensation is lost over the radial two-thirds of the palm as well as the thumb, index finger and radial half of the middle finger. A more proximal injury results in loss of pronation of the forearm and a weakening of wrist flexion.

Answer 3

(8) This is likely to be a supra-condylar fracture. It is important that a careful neurovascular examination is carried out due to the risk of damage to the median and ulnar nerves, as well as the brachial artery.

Answer 4

(2) Destruction of soft tissues is seen in patients with rheumatoid arthritis not osteoarthritis.

Answer 5

(1) The coracoid process is found in the shoulder joint and is the site of attachment for several important structures.

Self-assessment

ANSWERS TO HAND AND WRIST QUESTIONS

Answer 1
(6) **Mallet finger**. The history describes a typical mechanism of injury for Mallet finger. The examination findings are also consistent with the deformity produced by rupture of the extensor tendon in the distal portion of the finger, so this is the correct answer.

Answer 2
(8) **Scaphoid fracture**. If a patient has the clinical signs of a scaphoid fracture, you must treat as if it is this, even if you cannot see a fracture on x-ray. This is because scaphoid fractures are often difficult to detect on x-ray immediately after the injury, and may only become apparent on subsequent follow up x-rays. However, the risk of non-union and avascular necrosis of the scaphoid remains, and so this patient must be treated appropriately with close follow up to reduce the risk of these complications in the event that she does have a fractured scaphoid bone.

Answer 3
(4) **Dupuytren's disease**. This patient is describing a fixed flexion deformity of his right ring finger, a sign of Dupuytren's disease. The relevance of his father having the same condition is that the disease is often familial. It may also be known as Dupuytren's contracture.

Answer 4
(1) **Durkin's test**. Although Tinel's and Phalen's are valid tests for carpal tunnel syndrome, Durkin's has been described as the most sensitive for the disease. Finkelstein's test is for de Quervain's disease and the Ortolani test evaluates hip dislocation in infants.

Answer 5
(5) **Trigger finger**. This patient has signs consistent with trigger finger in his left ring finger. The significance of the patient having diabetes mellitus is that it is a risk factor for the disease.

ANSWERS TO SACRUM AND PELVIS QUESTIONS

Answer 1
(2) **Ankylosing spondylitis**. This patient has presented with features typical of ankylosing spondylitis and so this is a differential that needs to be explored.

Answer 2
(9) Tuberculosis. This man presented with symptoms of TB, which also appears to be involving his left sacroiliac joint. Appropriate investigations need to be carried out and treatment administered if he tests positive for the disease. Close contacts will also need to be tested for the disease.

Answer 3
(6) Osteomalacia. This condition is commonly caused by an adequate intake of vitamin D, which can occur in strict vegetarians or vegans, or in people who are not exposed to enough sunlight. Because of this, this woman needs to be investigated to see whether she has the disease, and supplementary vitamin D given if necessary.

Answer 4
(1) Osteoarthritis. Acetabular fractures are commonly associated with osteoarthritis as a complication. Often the osteoarthritis is treated by hip replacement. In a RTA like the one described above, the femur is likely to also be fractured. Posterior dislocation of the hip is also sustained by the method of injury described above and is associated with osteoarthritis.

Answer 5
(1) Digital rectal examination. If this patient has a urethral injury the prostate is likely to be high-riding on DRE and the patient will not be able to pass urine. Discussion with a senior doctor will need to take place about whether to try passing a catheter or not in a patient like this as this may cause further injury to the urethra.

ANSWERS TO HIP QUESTIONS

Answer 1
(2) Barlow's manoeuvre. This is a paediatric orthopaedic test to check for developmental dysplasia of the hip joint. A positive test indicates that the hip joint can be dislocated when pressure is applied to the hip joint (developmental dysplasia of the hip (DDH)).

Answer 2
(3) DEXA. Elderly females are particularly at risk of developing osteoporosis. This is due to insufficient levels of oestrogen after the menopause. Bone density is decreased which increases the risk of a bone fracture if they fall. This patient has risk factors and so the chances of sustaining a neck of femur (NOF) fracture are even greater. A DEXA scan measures bone mineral density.

Answer 3

(9) Thomas' test. The test is used to examine for fixed flexion deformity of the hip. The first part of the test involves 'obliterating' the pelvic tilt by flexing both hips. This compensates for a hip flexion deformity by neutralizing lumbar lordosis and stabilizes the pelvis prior to extending one leg back to the couch.

Answer 4

(4) Psoas. The origin of the psoas muscle is from the transverse processes of L1-4. It is inserted into the lesser trochanter of the femur. Psoas is a flexor and internal rotator of the hip joint. In hip fracture, it becomes an external rotator due to loss of the normal hip fulcrum.

Answer 5

(1) 0–30°. This is the normal range of movement of hip adduction. Remember, the pelvis needs to be fixed by crossing the patient's legs.

ANSWERS TO KNEE QUESTIONS

Answer 1

(6) Osteochondritis dissecans. This condition affects those in the teens and early 20s. It is important that a correct diagnosis is made in these cases as if missed then the segment will not heal and the patient is likely to return many years down the line with osteoarthritis (OA) of the knee. Meniscal tear could be considered but the lack of locking and intermittent swelling do not fit with this.

Answer 2

(8) This man has a popliteal aneurysm. The foot drop is caused by the expansile mass putting pressure on the peroneal nerve. It is vital that this man is also investigated for the presence of an abdominal aortic aneurysm as they commonly occur together. Many cases are bilateral, therefore always check the other leg.

Answer 3

(1) This is a typical history for an ACL tear. Although the clinical special tests are important, they are often unable to be done in the acute setting as the patient's quadriceps and hamstring muscles contract following the injury. Combined with the pain that the patient is in, it is often very difficult to accurately assess the ligaments. The haemarthrosis develops as a result of the torn structures. In any patient with an ACL injury, it is important to look for other associated injuries such as a meniscal tear or medial collateral ligament damage.

Answer 4

(1) A deep trochlear groove. A deep trochlear groove is an important restraint on the patella, particularly a high lateral wall which will reduce the chance of the patella being displaced laterally. Conversely, a shallow trochlear groove is a risk factor for recurrent dislocation.

Answer 5

(4) The medial meniscus can be easily damaged with a twisting force as seen in this case. It would be important to assess the integrity of all the ligaments supporting the knee, but the clue in the history is the locking. This occurs when a loose flap or segment of the meniscus is caught in the joint preventing further movement. The knee should not be forced to move but will often unlock itself after a brief period of time.

ANSWERS TO ANKLE AND FOOT QUESTIONS

Answer 1

(7) Plantarflex. Simmond's test is used to diagnose whether the Achilles tendon is intact. If the tendon has ruptured and the calf is squeezed while the patient is prone then the foot will remain still. If the Achilles is intact, the foot will plantarflex. To determine normal for that patient, always compare sides.

Answer 2

(3) Equinovarus. In club foot, the foot points downwards and is turned inwards. In a third of cases both feet are affected. There is a male:female ratio of 2:1.

Answer 3

(6) Invert. The anterior talofibular ligament is one of the three lateral ligaments of the ankle. The origin is the lateral malleolus. The insertion is into the talus hence the name talofibular. It is commonly injured when the foot is forcefully inverted.

Answer 4

(4) IV. Salter-Harris classification type IV ankle fracture in a child.

Answer 5

(1) Calcaneal tenderness. The Ottawa ankle and foot rules are very useful in excluding an ankle or foot fracture and avoid unnecessary x-ray examinations. Navicular tenderness was not included and would be an indication for an x-ray.

21 Rheumatology

RHEUMATOID ARTHRITIS QUESTIONS

In each of the following clinical situations, you must choose the most likely diagnosis. Each option may be used once, more than once or not at all.

DIAGNOSTIC OPTIONS:

1. Episcleritis
2. Glaucoma
3. ↓ Hb, ↓ platelets, ↑ leukocytes
4. Interleukin-2
5. Interleukin-7
6. ↓ leukocytes, ↑ platelets, ↓ Hb
7. ↓ leukocytes, ↓platelets, ↓ Hb
8. Maculopathy
9. Retinitis
10. Tumour necrosis factor-α

Question 1

You are the junior doctor in a rheumatology clinic. The specialist nurse is busy with patients, and the senior doctor has just diagnosed a woman with rheumatoid arthritis (RA). The patient is a scientist and wants to know the pathology behind the disease. The doctor has asked you to explain it to her. During your consultation she asks what cytokines are involved, you discuss one with her.

Question 2

You are the rheumatologist in clinic one afternoon. You are looking through the notes of the next patient waiting to be seen. At their last appointment, you suspected they had rheumatoid arthritis and so ordered some tests including a full blood count (FBC). You have the results of the FBC in front of you and it shows results that would be likely to be seen in a patient with RA.

Question 3

You are the doctor in a general ophthalmology clinic. The next patient to see has been referred by a rheumatologist. The patient is a man with RA who is suspected to have developed an ocular feature of RA. After seeing the patient you agree with the rheumatologist that the patient has in fact developed this disease.

Question 4

A 61-year-old woman has suffered from RA for 19 years. She is on appropriate treatment for her disease, but unfortunately it is severe and has caused deformities of her hands. She has difficulties doing activities of daily living, such as washing and dressing. Choose the single most likely deformity you would see in this woman's hands:

1. Distal interphalangeal joint swelling
2. Knuckle subluxation
3. Radial deviation of the fingers
4. T-shaped thumb
5. Ulnar deviation of the wrist

Question 5

A 55 year old man has recently been diagnosed with RA. His rheumatologist has prescribed him a steroid and a non-steroidal anti-inflammatory drug (NSAID). Symptoms remain troublesome. What other medication is likely to be helpful? From the list below, choose the drug that the doctor is most likely to prescribe the patient for his RA.

1. Acyclovir
2. Amlodipine
3. Methotrexate
4. Rituximab
5. Simvastatin

CRYSTAL ARTHROPATHIES QUESTIONS

For each of the following clinical scenarios, all of which focus on the crystal arthropathies, choose the most likely answer. Each option may be used once, more than once or not at all.

Options:

1. Acute gout
2. Allopurinol
3. Chronic gout
4. Fifth metatarsophalangeal (MTP) joint
5. First MTP joint
6. Intra-articular steroid injection
7. Knee
8. Negatively birefringent
9. Positively birefringent
10. Pseudogout
11. Septic arthritis
12. Thiazide diuretic

QUESTION 1

Your next patient at a GP practice is known to have recently suffered their third episode of gout in the past year and you decide that they require prophylactic treatment. What treatment would be appropriate?

Question 2

A 55-year-old male carpenter presents to the Emergency Department with a hot painful swollen left knee. He denies any trauma but does mention that he has recently forgotten to wear his knee pads at work. On examination, the man looks unwell and has a temperature of 37.9°C. What diagnosis must you exclude first?

Question 3

A 60-year-old woman presents with a hot swollen right knee. An x-ray reveals chondrocalcinosis of the meniscus. You diagnose pseudogout. You have also aspirated the knee and sent this to the laboratory to be analysed which has confirmed the presence of crystals. Under polarized light, how are these likely to appear?

Question 4

Which of the following is not recommended as a treatment in acute gout?
1. Allopurinol
2. Colchicine
3. Intra-articular steroid injection
4. NSAIDs
5. Hydrocortisone

Question 5

Which of the following conditions is not associated with pseudogout?
1. Haemochromatosis
2. Hypercalcaemia
3. Hyperkalaemia
4. Hypomagnesaemia
5. Hypothyroidism

DIFFUSE CONNECTIVE TISSUE DISEASES QUESTIONS

For each of the following questions, all of which focus on diffuse connective tissue diseases, choose the most likely answer. Each option may be used once, more than once or not at all.

DIAGNOSTIC OPTIONS:

1. Reactive arthritis
2. Multiple myeloma
3. Chronic fatigue syndrome
4. Systemic lupus erythematosus (SLE)
5. Fibromyalgia
6. Sjögren's syndrome
7. Lymphoma
8. Vasculitis
9. Polymyositis
10. Rheumatoid arthritis

Self-assessment

Question 1

A 65-year-old man presents to his GP with a new onset cough and feeling generally unwell over the past 2 days. On taking a history, the GP elicits that the patient was in hospital about a year ago after he presented to Accident and Emergency with muscle pains, increased fatigue on walking, and pyrexia. He had a course of prednisolone but he cannot remember what the doctors said was wrong. What was the most likely diagnosis?

Question 2

A 50-year-old woman presents to her GP with pain all over her body. She says that she gets a burning pain over various points of her body that are worse on palpation and she has been more tired than usual recently. On further questioning, the patient says that she has been feeling quite 'low' recently as she recently split up from her husband and she is under a great deal of stress at work. The GP does some tests but they all come back normal. What is the most likely diagnosis?

Question 3

A 45-year-old woman presents to the rheumatology clinic. She complains of dry, gritty eyes, a dry mouth and painful joints. You suspect Sjögren's syndrome and want to test lacrimal gland function. Which test is most appropriate from the list below?

1. Erythrocyte sedimentation rate (ESR) level
2. Rose Bengal staining
3. Schirmer's test
4. Test for antinuclear antibodies (ANA)
5. Test for Anti-Ro antibodies

Question 4

A 30-year-old woman presents to her GP. She has recently been diagnosed with systemic lupus erythematosus after presenting with weight loss, fatigue, anaemia, arthritis, and a facial rash a couple of months previously. She is a biologist and wants to know the pathology behind the disease. She read somewhere that there is an increase in activity of a certain type of cell. Which cells is she referring to?

1. Neutrophils
2. T cells
3. B cells
4. Macrophages
5. Erythrocytes.

SPONDYLOARTHRITIDES QUESTIONS

For each of the following questions choose the most likely answer. Each option may be used once, more than once or not at all.

DIAGNOSTIC OPTIONS:

1. Aortitis
2. Conjunctivitis
3. Dactylitis
4. Enthesitis
5. Episcleritis

6. Folliculitis
7. Psoriasis
8. Sacroilitis
9. Urethritis
10. Vasculitis

Question 1

A 23-year-old man attends the Emergency Department complaining of a 5-day history of left knee pain and itchy red eyes. He denies any trauma. On examination, he has a swollen, red, tender left knee; epiphoreic eyes with red sclerae. What other inflammatory condition is this patient likely to have that he has not included in his history?

Question 2

A dermatology patient is referred to your rheumatology clinic. Your colleague is concerned about the patient's progressive joint swelling that affects the hands and the right ankle with an associated rash in the extensor surfaces. What kind of inflammation is this?

Question 3

Mr Beaumont is a 20-year-old man who has been referred to you by his GP who was concerned about his patient's progressive back stiffness. On examination, the patient has reduced range of all spinal movements. You take a blood sample for tissue typing which shows HLA-B27. What condition is causing the symptoms?

Question 4

A 30-year-old male with late-stage ankylosing spondylitis presents to his GP. The surgery contacts you to discuss various treatment options as 'his spine has become worse'. Before discussing medication, you go online to look at his latest outpatient spinal x-ray. You point out to the GP that the patient's x-ray reveals bone changes that more likely than not are causing the back symptoms. What are diagnostic radiographic changes may be seen?

1. Osteophytes
2. Stenoses

3. Subluxations
4. Syndesmophytes
5. Wedge fractures

Question 5

A 46-year-old patient attends your rheumatology clinic for a three-month follow up appointment. He has longstanding anklosing spondylitis. You are already treating him with NSAIDs. Unfortunately, you see that the patient has deteriorated and you need to take the next step in medical treatment. What is the drug of choice?
1. Codeine phosphate
2. Etanercept
3. Methotrexate
4. Osteotomy
5. Sulphasalazine.

NON-INFLAMMATORY ARTHROSES QUESTIONS

For each of the following questions, choose the most likely answer. The options can be used once, more than once or not at all.

DIAGNOSTIC OPTIONS:

1. Arthoscopy
2. Exercise
3. Hydrotherapy
4. Intra-articular injection
5. Joint replacement
6. NSAIDs
7. Oral steroids
8. Paracetamol
9. Transcutaneous electrical nerve stimulation (TENS)
10. Thermotherapy

Question 1

You are observing a general practitioner clinic. A wheelchair-bound 78-year-old woman presents with longstanding osteoarthritis (OA) of both knees which is being treated with simple analgesia. She has a past medical history of peptic ulcers and would like advice on how to ease her knee pain. What does the GP recommend?

Question 2

A 45-year-old former rugby league professional presents at your orthopaedic clinic complaining of a 'clicking' sound and pain on moving his right knee. He has been taking 'painkillers' for four years. The pain is increasing and he has stopped running. On examination, he has marked crepitus and locking on flexion and extension of the right knee. What treatment would you recommend?

Question 3

A 70-year-old female patient presents at the clinic complaining of left hip pain and not walking 'properly'. You examine the patient and find her to be obese (body mass index (BMI) of 32), but no other significant clinical findings. X-ray reveals minimal loss of space in the left hip joint. What would be your first recommendation in managing this patient?

Question 4

A 50-year-old man presents to the orthopaedic clinic complaining of a dull ache over his right hip and groin that has been getting worse over the last couple of weeks. He fell over onto his right side a few months ago but managed the resulting pain with over-the counter-analgesia; however, it seems to have worsened recently and is now affecting his mobility. On taking a full history, you find out he has been taking steroids for severe asthma intermittently for most of his life, and his recent course has been for about a year. What disease do you need to exclude in this patient?

1. Osteoarthritis
2. Osteonecrosis
3. Referred hip pain
4. Septic arthritis
5. Urinary tract infection

Question 5

During your medical school finals, you have to complete a rheumatology pictures OSCE (objective structured clinical examination) station. You are examining an x-ray showing a swelling on the index finger affecting the proximal interphalangeal (PIP) joint. What is this nodal phenomenon?

1. Bouchard's node
2. Boutonnière deformity
3. Heberden's node
4. Palmar erythema
5. Swan neck deformity.

DISORDERS OF BONE METABOLISM: OSTEOPOROSIS QUESTIONS

For each of the following clinical scenarios, all of which focus on osteoporosis, choose the most likely answer. Each option may be used once, more than once or not at all.

DIAGNOSTIC OPTIONS:

1. Coeliac disease
2. Crohn's disease
3. Early menopause
4. Glucocorticoid-induced osteoporosis
5. Hyperparathyroidism
6. Multiple myeloma
7. Osteonecrosis of the jaw
8. Post-menopausal osteoporosis
9. Secondary osteoporosis
10. Vitamin D deficiency

Question 1

Your next patient has been referred to see you as she sustained her first ever fracture having tripped over a step. She is 70 and went through the menopause aged 52 years. She has been receiving treatment for polymyalgia rheumatica over the past five months, but insists she takes no other medication. She is otherwise fit and well. What has most likely contributed to this woman's fracture?

Question 2

During a normal work up of a patient with suspected osteoporosis, you find positive results of tests for endomysial antibodies and anti-tissue transglutaminase antibodies. What underlying diagnosis may be causing their osteoporosis?

Question 3

A 68-year-old woman stumbles while hurrying for a bus and falls awkwardly landing on her side. In the Emergency Department, examination reveals that her right leg is shortened and externally rotated and she is unable to walk. From her history, you note that she had a hysterectomy and bilateral oophrectomy at the age of 35. X-rays confirm a broken hip. What is the most likely cause for this woman's apparent reduced bone density.

Question 4

Which of the following is not an instruction for when taking bisphosphonates?
1. Ensure that you do not take the tablet on an empty stomach
2. Sit upright or stand up for at least 30 minutes after taking the tablet
3. Take your tablet in the morning
4. Take the tablet with a full glass of tap water
5. Wait at least 1 hour before taking any other tablets

Question 5

Which of the following conditions is not a risk factor for developing osteoporosis?
1. Anorexia
2. Diabetes mellitus

3. Hypothyroidism
4. Multiple myeloma
5. Rheumatoid arthritis

DISORDERS OF BONE METABOLISM: OSTEROMALACIA AND RICKETS QUESTIONS

For each of the following clinical scenarios, all of which focus on osteromalacia, choose the most likely answer. Each option may be used once, more than once or not at all.

DIAGNOSTIC OPTIONS:

1. Tuberculosis
2. Marfan syndrome
3. Paget's disease
4. Osteoarthritis
5. Osteomalacia

6. Osteomyelitis
7. Rheumatoid arthritis
8. Rickets
9. Osteopenia
10. Bone metastases

Question 1

A 30-year-old woman from the Middle East attends an appointment at your clinic in a GP surgery. She complains of back pain that has been present for some time now. There is no history of trauma, but you do note she is wearing a burka and is a vegetarian. What disease do you need to investigate for?

Question 2

A mother brings her eight-month-old daughter into the GP at which you are working. She is worried that her child's head looks a different shape to other children at the playgroup she attends. She has also noticed that the child's wrists are swollen. You have a look at the 'red book' the mother has helpfully brought along, and note that the growth chart shows the child has been between the 2nd and 0.4th centiles since birth. On further questioning, you discover that the family are strict vegans and the mother has not been out with the baby much due to post-natal depression. What disease would you suspect this child has?

DISORDERS OF BONE METABOLISM: PAGET'S DISEASE QUESTIONS

For each of the following questions, all of which focus on Paget's disease, choose the most likely answer. Each option may be used once, more than once or not at all.

DIAGNOSTIC OPTIONS

1. ↓ action of osteoclasts
2. ↑ action of osteoclasts
3. ↑ action of osteocytes
4. Fine trabeculation
5. Hypercalcaemia
6. Hyperkalaemia
7. Hypernatraemia
8. Hypocalcaemia
9. Sclerosis
10. Thin bones

Question 1

You are a junior doctor in a general practice. Mrs Pagète has an appointment for your morning surgery. She comes to see you for a medication review and mentions that she has recently been diagnosed with Paget's disease. However, she does not understand what this is apart from that her bones are affected. What is the pathogenesis behind her disease?

Question 2

You are a junior doctor teaching some medical students about Paget's disease. One student asks what changes are seen on x-rays of patients with Paget's disease. You explain that it depends on the stage of the disease, but show them an x-ray of an abnormality that is commonly seen later in the disease. What was it?

Question 3

Mr Clast is a patient who is currently under investigation for Paget's disease. You are his GP and he has come to see you because he is anxious to know more about the disease, in particular the complications. You start by explaining one to him, which one did you tell him about?

Question 4

A 65-year-old man has suffered from Paget's disease for ten years. He is on appropriate treatment for the disease and has regular appointments to make sure the disease is being adequately controlled. He has a blood test at these appointments to measure something which is important to monitor in patients with Paget's as it indicates the level of activity of the disease. What does this blood test measure?

1. Full blood count
2. Liver function
3. Serum alkaline phosphatase
4. Thyroid function
5. Urea and electrolytes

Question 5

A 60-year-old man has recently been diagnosed with Paget's disease. The doctor is now considering what regular medications to prescribe him. He decides on a drug, which one does he choose?

1. Alendronic acid
2. Methotrexate
3. Prednisolone
4. Simvastatin
5. Teriparatide.

BONE AND JOINT INFECTION QUESTIONS

For each of the following clinical scenarios, choose the most likely diagnosis. Each option may be used once, more than once or not at all.

DIAGNOSTIC OPTIONS:

1. Bone metastases
2. Gout
3. Lymphoma
4. Osteomyelitis
5. Osteonecrosis
6. Paget's disease
7. Pseudogout
8. Septic arthritis
9. Sjögren's syndrome
10. Tuberculosis

Question 1

A 25-year-old intravenous drug user (IVDU) presents to the minor injuries unit with an erythematous, swollen and painful right thigh. On examination, you notice the patient is pyrexial, there are track marks from where the patient has injected drugs into her thigh, a number of small abscesses are present in her thigh, and she has marked tenderness on palpation of the femur. What disease do you need to exclude in this patient?

Question 2

A 61-year-old man presents with an acutely inflamed, tender knee that is warm to the touch and very painful to mobilize. He is feverish and has a pyrexia of 38°C. He underwent a knee arthroscopy 10 days ago for a bothersome meniscal tear. One of the arthroscopic port sites is erythematous and producing a small amount of discharge. Blood tests reveal a raised C-reactive protein (CRP) and white cell count (WCC).

BONE TUMOURS QUESTIONS

For each of the following clinical scenarios, choose the most likely diagnosis. Each option may be used once, more than once or not at all.

DIAGNOSTIC OPTIONS:

1. Bone metastases
2. Dermatomyositis
3. Fibromyalgia
4. Lymphoma
5. Multiple myeloma
6. Osteoarthritis
7. Osteomalacia
8. Paget's disease
9. Rickets
10. Sjögren's syndrome

Question 1:

A 75-year-old man presents to the osteoporosis clinic. He recently sustained a fragility fracture. On further questioning, he admits to being more tired recently and has suffered several recent chest infections. As part of his work up, his urine was tested which was positive for Bence Jones protein. What is the diagnosis?

Question 2

You are the junior doctor working in general practice. A 60-year-old woman comes to see you complaining of back pain which has been troubling her for a couple of months. She has no history of trauma, but has been in remission from breast cancer for three years. What is the most likely diagnosis?

ANSWERS TO RHEUMATOID ARTHRITIS QUESTIONS

Answer 1

(10) Tumour necrosis factor-α. This cytokine and interleukin-1 are the two most important cytokines in the pathogenesis of rheumatoid arthritis.

Answer 2

(6) ↓ leukocytes, ↑ platelets, ↓ Hb. This is the most likely FBC profile you would see in a patient with RA from the choices given. Anaemia is a common occurrence in RA, platelets are often raised, and the leukopenia can be due to an extra-articular feature of RA: Felty's syndrome, where splenomegaly would also be present.

Answer 3

(1) Episcleritis. Keratoconjunctivitis, scleritis and episcleritis are all extra-articular features of RA. The other ocular answers on the list: glaucoma, maculopathy and retinitis, are all possible diseases of the eye this patient could have, but they are not features of RA itself, they have different causes.

Answer 4

(2) Knuckle subluxation. This is the most likely change to be seen in this woman's hands because none of the other changes on the list occur in RA. Changes in the hand that are seen in RA include ulnar deviation of the fingers, radial deviation of the wrist, Z-shaped thumb, boutonnière and/or swan neck deformity of the fingers, and wrist subluxation. RA does not involve the distal interphalangeal joints.

Answer 5

(3) Methotrexate. Rheumatologists often initially prescribe an NSAID, a steroid (e.g. prednisolone) and a disease modifying anti-rheumatic drug (DMARD) for the treatment of RA. This patient is already taking an NSAID and a steroid, so the most likely drug to be prescribed from the list next is a DMARD, methotrexate. Rituximab is a drug used in the treatment of RA, but it is only usually used when other treatments have failed to work. None of the other drugs on the list would be appropriate treatments for RA.

ANSWERS TO CRYSTAL ARTHROPATHIES QUESTIONS

Answer 1

(2) Allopurinol. This is the first-line choice for the treatment of chronic gout. It is important to remember when prescribing this that it may precipitate an episode of acute gout and therefore it is necessary to wait 1–2 weeks after an acute attack before starting the allopurinol.

Answer 2

(11) An important possible diagnosis here is septic arthritis. The knee aspirate is likely to show yellow pus.

Answer 3

(9) Positively birefringent. Pseudogout crystals are weakly positively birefringent and are rhomboid in shape. This is in contrast to gout crystals which are strongly negatively birefringent and needle-shaped.

Answer 4

(1) Allopurinol must not be prescribed for the management of acute gout. Its role is in prophylaxis of acute gouty episodes and complications of hyperuricaemia. It may trigger an acute attack of gout. Therefore, 1–2 weeks must pass following an acute episode of gout before allopurinol is started.

Answer 5

(3) Hyperkalaemia (raised serum potassium level) is not associated with pseudogout or gout. If severe, it is a medical emergency as potentially fatal arrhythmias may develop.

ANSWERS TO DIFFUSE CONNECTIVE TISSUE DISEASES QUESTIONS

Answer 1
(9) Polymyositis. The combination of muscle pains, increased fatigue on walking and pyrexia treated with steroids suggests that this patient could have been diagnosed with polymyositis. The fact he now presents with a cough and feeling unwell could suggest that he has aspiration pneumonia as this disease can affect the respiratory muscles.

Answer 2
(5) Fibromyalgia. The patient describes symptoms that occur in fibromyalgia. The disease is often triggered by depression which this patient appears to have. The fact that no abnormalities have been found on tests increases the likelihood that this is the diagnosis.

Answer 3
(3) Schirmer's test. All of the tests listed are appropriate to carry out in a patient with suspected Sjögren's syndrome, but Schirmer's test is the only one listed that assesses tear production.

Answer 4
(3) B cells. In systemic lupus erythematosus, there is dysfunction of the immune system with increased activity of B cells.

ANSWERS TO SPONDYLOARTHRITIDES QUESTIONS

Answer 1
(9) Urethritis. The likely diagnosis is reactive arthritis which is more common in young men. The triad of arthritis, conjunctivitis and urethritis can be remembered by 'can't see, can't pee, can't climb up a tree'.

Answer 2
(7) Psoriasis. You should be suspicious of psoriatic arthritis when a patient presents with oligoarthritis and has a rash. Psoriasis affects the extensor skin surfaces particularly the posterior elbow and anterior knee (not to be confused with eczema which has a flexor distribution).

Answer 3

(8) Sacroilitis. HLA-B27 is the histocompatibility antigen that has a strong association with spondyloarthritides, particularly ankylosing spondylitis.

Answer 4

(4) Syndesmophytes. Patients with ankylosing spondylitis are particularly susceptible to developing syndesmophytes. These are vertical bony outgrowths in the spinal ligaments from the intervertebral joints. This eventually leads to spinal fusion and on x-ray a 'bamboo spine' appearance.

Answer 5

(2) Etanercept. A rheumatologist's first line of pharmacological treatment is usually to prescribe patients with an NSAID. This patient has already had this treatment. Tumour necrosis factor-α blockers are reserved for when other medication has failed but may be dramatically effective.

ANSWERS TO NON-INFLAMMATORY ARTHROSES QUESTIONS

Answer 1

(9) TENS. This can help with pain relief and offers possible minor local muscle conditioning around the knee for a patient who has diminished mobility. NSAIDs are contraindicated because of the patient's history of peptic ulceration and at risk age group for gastrointestinal (GI) bleed. Intra-articular injection is not indicated unless the patient has no benefit from TENS and oral analgesia.

Answer 2

(1) Arthroscopy. The patient is 45 years old. He has had a career in a high impact sport and would be vulnerable to early onset OA. Arthroscopy would detect and remove loose bodies and return the knee to reasonable function. Joint replacement is not a first option at such a young age.

Answer 3

(2) Exercise. This is a major component of all weight loss programmes and is to be encouraged irrespective of the age of the patient or the severity of the OA. Exercise should be incorporated into the patient's daily life.

Answer 4

(2) Osteonecrosis. This patient has had right hip and groin pain since falling on to his right side a few months ago. There is a high likelihood he has fractured his right hip and the fact he has been taking steroids for a long period of time increases the risk of this. The fracture could have disrupted the blood supply to the femoral head, causing osteonecrosis.

Answer 5

(1) Bouchard's node. The picture is highlighting a Bouchard's node on the PIP of the index finger. This is a diagnostic hand sign of osteoarthritis.

ANSWERS TO DISORDERS OF BONE METABOLISM: OSTEOPOROSIS QUESTIONS

Answer 1

(4) Glucocorticoid-induced osteoporosis. Although this patient may well have post-menopausal osteoporosis, the key factor in this case is the treatment with glucocorticoids for polymyalgia rheumatica. Glucocorticoids are a cause of secondary osteoporosis and so patients should be treated with a bisphosphonate, calcium and vitamin D supplement when they commence oral glucocorticoid therapy which is likely to last over three months.

Answer 2

(1) Coeliac disease. Endomysial antibodies and anti-tissue transglutaminase antibodies are important markers for coeliac disease. Coeliac disease is a gluten-sensitive enteropathy. If patients adhere to a gluten-free diet, their bone density is likely to improve, although they may still require bisphosphonate therapy. A diagnosis of coeliac disease can be confirmed on jejunal or distal duodenal biopsy which may show villous atrophy.

Answer 3

(3) Early menopause. The average for menopause is 52 years. By having a total hysterectomy, this woman has had an early menopause. It would be important to ask her about hormone replacement therapy. As she has sustained a fragility fracture, it would be important for this patient to have a bone DXA (dual energy x-ray absorptiometry) scan and careful history taken to determine whether this patient has osteoporosis.

Answer 4

(1) Ensure that you do not take the tablet on an empty stomach. It is important that bisphosphonate treatments are taken on an empty stomach. There is a long list of careful instructions which must be followed to ensure maximal bioavailability of the medication, while minimizing the risk of gastric irritation. Due to the high affinity of bisphosphonates for calcium, it is vital the tablets are taken on an empty stomach with tap water to prevent the bisphosphonate binding to calcium in food contents before it is absorbed into the bloodstream.

Answer 5

(3) Hypothyroidism. Hypothyroidism is not a risk factor; it is the high levels of thyroid hormone which may cause osteoporosis. This is because hyperthyroidism increases the rate of bone turnover with insufficient new bone formation. This results in a net loss of bone and an increased risk of fracture. Patients with hypothyroidism are only at an increased risk of osteoporosis if they are given too much thyroxine replacement which will result in increased bone turnover.

ANSWERS TO DISORDERS OF BONE METABOLISM: OSTEOMALACIA AND RICKETS QUESTIONS

Answer 1

(5) Osteomalacia. The history of back pain is rather vague in this question, but the mention of a burka being worn by the patient and her vegetarian diet would raise your suspicion of the bone pain being due to osteomalacia due to inadequate vitamin D. Since the patient is 30 years old she does not have rickets.

Answer 2

(8) Rickets. The child has clinical features suggestive of rickets which include frontal bossing, swollen wrists and growth problems. The fact the family are strict vegans and that the child has not been out much suggests the child is not getting an adequate intake of vitamin D for bone mineralization. Osteomalacia would be a good answer in an adult with similar problems and in this case it may be vigilant to investigate the mother for this disease.

ANSWERS TO DISORDERS OF BONE METABOLISM: PAGET'S DISEASE QUESTIONS

Answer 1

(2) ↑ action of osteoclasts. In Paget's disease, osteoclasts resorb bone at a higher rate than in normal subjects. This is the only answer on the list which describes the pathogenesis of Paget's disease.

Answer 2

(9) Sclerosis. This is often a late feature found on x-rays of patients with Paget's disease. Other features seen on x-rays of patients with the disease include thickened bone and coarse trabeculation.

Answer 3

(5) Hypercalcaemia. This is a known complication of Paget's disease and is an important electrolyte imbalance to consider. Hypernatraemia, hyperkalaemia and hypocalcaemia are not associated with Paget's disease.

Answer 4

(3) Serum alkaline phosphatase. In patients with Paget's disease, it is important that this is monitored regularly. The other blood tests listed are all important, but only serum alkaline phosphatase will reveal the level of activity of Paget's disease in a patient.

Answer 5

(1) Alendronic acid. This is a bisphosphonate which may improve some of the symptoms associated with Paget's disease. None of the other listed medications would be suitable for the treatment of Paget's disease.

ANSWERS TO BONE AND JOINT INFECTION QUESTIONS

Answer 1

(9) Osteomyelitis needs to be excluded in this patient. The patient is at risk of developing osteomyelitis as there is evidence she injects into her right thigh and there are small abscesses present, suggesting she is using dirty needles. Often IVDU will also be malnourished and could have immunosuppressive diseases, such as HIV, putting them more at risk of getting osteomyelitis.

Answer 2

(2) Septic arthritis is high on your list of differentials in this case. There is a clear source of infection that appears to have tracked into the joint. The most likely organism is *Staphyloccus aureus*. A joint aspirate needs to be taken and sent for microscopy, culture and sensitivity (MC&S) and broad spectrum intravenous antibiotics should be commenced.

ANSWERS TO BONE TUMOURS QUESTIONS

Answer 1

(5) Multiple myeloma. Suspicion for this disease should first be raised on identification that this man fractured his humerus from a low impact force. In this patient, appropriate investigations were carried out, one of which showed Bence Jones proteins in the urine which is characteristic of multiple myeloma.

Answer 2

(1) Bone metastases. This woman has a history of breast cancer. Even though she is in remission, her back pain is likely to be due to bone metastases from the primary breast cancer. Always have a high index of suspicion when a patient with a current or previous malignancy presents to you with bone pain.

Index